Your Beautiful Trauma

A practical guide to help you
convert crisis into full-scale transformation

Emi Garzitto (PhD)

ISBN-13: 978-0-9988546-5-6
ISBN-10: 0-9988546-5-4

Published by: Celebrity Expert Author
http://celebrityexpertauthor.com

Canadian Address:	US Address:
1108 - 1155 The High Street,	1300 Boblett Street
Coquitlam, BC, Canada	Unit A-218
V3B.7W4	Blaine, WA 98230
Phone: (604) 941-3041	Phone: (866) 492-6623
Fax: (604) 944-7993	Fax: (250) 493-6603

Contents

Prologue

A thousand mile journey begins with one step.

Lao Tse

Your work has downsized and you are escorted out of the building.

Your dream home goes into foreclosure.

Your husband leaves you.

A major car accident leaves you paralyzed.

You have been told you have terminal cancer.

You cannot pull yourself out of bed for the third straight day.

Your crisis begins.

THIS IS YOUR HANDBOOK on crisis. It will provide you with the necessary tools to help you navigate through the circumstances in your life that have left you feeling broken and lost. This book will provide suggestions, support and encouragement to help you in those moments where you might feel abandoned, defeated and alone. This is about helping you find the strength, the courage and the wisdom that will take you to your real self. What I mean by your "real self" is the you that is comfortable in your own skin. It is not the perfect self; rather it is the self that has the courage to walk towards the desires of your heart. It is the self that has the strength to acknowledge life's failures – to collapse and get up again. It is the self that has the wisdom to learn from all the experiences of life, both painful and blissful.

At some point in my life I have been a little bit of everything. I have a Philosophy of Education PhD. I studied conflict – I tried to answer the question, "Can't we all just get along?" I've facilitated hundreds of workshops that helped participants manage their big feelings or helped them get along with their family or coworkers. I have spent most of my life surrounded by children, although I could not have any of my own. I have worked in schools as a counsellor, a teacher and a vice principal.

I also have an Energy Medicine practice, where I combine several holistic approaches that support clients in their healing. Energy Medicine views the body as a fluid ecosystem that functions best when all of its parts are balanced and calm. This means that I work with the body as well as the body's energy, electricity and feelings to help clients feel better. Energy Medicine acknowledges the role that feelings, memories, dreams and beliefs play in a person's health and wellbeing.

I am going to be there for you as you walk through your crisis. I am going to help you understand how you got to your crisis. I can keep you company, I can point you in the general direction and I can suggest tools and strategies that will move you through the crisis. I will give you lots of ideas on how to make this better but I cannot do the work for you. That will be up to you.

This book will help you arrive home - your real Home. Whatever predicament you are in, you are not in this space by accident. Be patient because, in the end, reading this book and following the advice and the steps will be the fastest route to getting you back on track. We are going to take this journey through your crisis together. I promise, I will not leave you until we get to the other side. Are you ready?

Chapter One
Crisis

There is a crack in everything. That's how the light gets in.
Leonard Cohen

You are what you repeatedly do. **Aristotle**

Doing and Undoing Are the Same Work

MY MOTHER FIRST BEGAN to teach me to knit when I
was six years old. She would begin with a square. She cast
the first row with her swift, expert fingers. She carefully
showed me how to hold the needles with the yarn looped
in between my fingers. She pierced a loop, then wrapped an
additional loop, and miraculously created another stitch.
When it was my turn to knit, my mother would peer over
me, sometimes putting her hands over mine, guiding me

through the process until I learned with my hands, my eyes, my ears and with the rest of me. Later, I would know this process by instinct; by feel, by sense, and by spirit, but in the beginning, I was just trying my best to follow my mom's hands.

I would try to do the same thing as she did, but inevitably, I made mistakes. In knitting, an undo requires backtracking. It means taking apart both the good and bad stitches in order to move forward and repair the offending loop. I hated the idea of going backwards. As an eight-year-old this was a disaster – it felt like *I* was the mistake.

Sometimes mamma would scrutinize my mistake and miraculously, she would repair it. Hooray! I would be spared the undo. I often watched mom pull apart a section. How could she drop stitches, yes with frustration, yes with impatience, but nevertheless get it done? She never cried or held a despairing tantrum - which I admit happened to me on more than one occasion. My mother would say in her Italian dialect, "Fa e disfa e dut un lavora" – roughly translated it means, "Doing and undoing are the same work."

Even now, it is not uncommon for a knitting project that I'm tackling to remain untouched for months, as I refuse to tear apart the beautiful colours and patterns. I pout. I stubbornly refuse to face the undo and so, I remain frozen until I can come up with the courage to pull apart the project. It physically hurts.

Sometimes I call my mom to complain, but I only get the despairing proverb, "Fa e disfa e dut un lavora", in a tone of, "What's the problem? Did you expect to knit without ever undoing your knitting?"

Much later, as an adult, I would understand that taking care of my undos was not just for knitting. It was also the key to living my life. Life and knitting are full of undos, full of backward steps, full of tearing up the past, just to get to the learning. In Italian culture, the idea of doing and undoing as one continual circle of achievement and completion is practiced daily.

In our busy digital lives, it is easy to pretend that the undo can be averted. We type out words on our computers, cut and paste, do, undo, redo with the touch of buttons. We can somehow leave the good bits alone. We have the illusion that undos are easy, but like all things sacred, the undo is painful, dangerous work. Yet, it is the painful, dangerous work that leads to the transformation we all ache to receive.

What is Crisis?

Crisis is a painful, radical interruption that provides an opportunity for full-scale transformation. It is any circumstance or condition that stops you from the life that you have practiced. You can't pretend anymore that everything is the same. It can be personal or it can be collective. It can be about the realization that you no longer believe whatever story you grew up with, or put all your faith in, or it can be about the Civil War that moves you and millions around you, out of your homes.

Crisis is painful, because it is a form of amputation. You are severing a relationship that you have relied on for a long time. The severing can take many forms: someone you love has broken your trust, a loved one dies, you lose your faith in a belief, a government or yourself. What you once relied upon is now unpredictable and flawed.

Crisis is radical because it is far-reaching and all encompassing. It means that all of the connections in your life have somehow disconnected and it is now up to you to figure out how to reassemble them. Or perhaps, it is your work to find a completely new place to connect. You can no longer rely on your past to guide your present. There is no clearly marked road to follow. You are usually completely out of your comfort zone and everything feels unfamiliar. Foreign. Dangerous.

The usual signals that help you in decision making no longer apply, or appear to rely on a new rule book – one that you do not currently own. In fact, the usual signposts and signals that used to help you make decisions no longer work. You are not sure anymore what is safe and what is dangerous. It may feel as if your own spirit has failed you, or maybe, the God you served for so many years, has betrayed you. You are lost.

Your feelings will be disrupted. The ones you have tried the hardest to ignore, or the feelings that you pretend do not belong to you are the ones that will arise with the greatest force. You may feel frozen, or you may have an explosion of feelings that you cannot process. They will often feel terribly dangerous - grief, rage, wrath. Or maybe you will feel helpless, weak, and ashamed.

Every part of your life is somehow altered. It is the breaking of a promise that life would take care of you. Your ability to view your life as "normal" is over. It is the mother of all interruptions. How are you supposed to find your way home when everything you have relied on has been taken away? How do you find your way home when you are cold, naked and blind? If it is not a punishment, what is it?

The Great Undo

The truth is, the seeds of crisis are sown over a very long period of time. In fact, before your crisis begins, there are many smaller cracks and conflicts that come before the crisis. Every small crack alerts you of your coming crisis. These small cracks can happen to you individually, and they can also happen in groups. Countries and communities in crisis follow the same pattern as personal ones, only with greater force. Because of their sheer size and scale, they often take longer to change. Terrorism, war and revolutions are all examples of large-scale transitions that take place on a global scale. The shifts can take years, generations and lifetimes to unravel.

Your own personal crisis takes place over long periods of time, slowly building steam. It may feel like an explosion, but in reality, there were a series of small fuel leaks that contributed to the devastation. The knitting knots gather over small repeated twists and turns that do not receive attention.

My clients often report that their crisis hit them out of nowhere. They didn't see the divorce coming. They didn't see their child's drug addiction, or their husband's financial crisis, or the affair. Yet crisis comes to you in small gradual increments. The bankruptcy is sudden, but the groundwork for the bankruptcy took place years and generations prior to the radical disruption. Your beliefs around money and your beliefs around abundance brought you, over time, towards the bankruptcy. Spiritual and financial bankruptcies take years to happen.

There are many clues that will indicate that you are heading into crisis. We are very good at pretending everything is "okay". There are cover-ups or Band-Aid patches that help you carry on and act as if no radical change is required, so you move forward - with worry, but still not ready to make a change. You will work very hard not to notice or ignore the signposts and signals until it is too late. It is important to understand the role each of these signals play in setting the stage for your impending crisis. The more you understand each of these signposts, the better your chance of navigating and moving through your crisis. In some cases, you might even avert your crisis altogether.

Clues that your crisis is coming arrive in your repeated conflicts, in the repeated feelings that hurt, in your distractions and addictions and in your physical, mental and spiritual exhaustion.

Crisis Shows Up in Your Repeated Conflicts

My repeated conflicts

Growing up, conflict was very dangerous and painful. My views on right and wrong were closely linked to my spirituality. Being wrong meant being disconnected to God. Whenever conflict came up, I did everything I could to avoid it. I pretended it wasn't happening. I tried to make myself invisible, while secretly desperately desiring to be seen. I would hide my feelings, all the while feeling as though there was something wrong with me. Conflict meant that someone was a winner and someone was a loser. As a child, I felt like I always ended up on the loser side of conflict. It reinforced my belief that I was not worthy of love.

I am sure this is what sparked my fascination for feelings and conflict. I was trying to find a way to stand up and face my childhood battles. As part of my thesis research, I came across Dannon Parry's book *Warriors of the Heart:*

A handbook for Conflict Resolution. In his book, Parry describes conflict as, "An opportunity for intimacy." An opportunity for intimacy? How could conflict bring me closer to others? How could something so painful and dangerous hold the key to receiving what I was really aching for – deep connection and understanding? Parry's words invited me to see conflict as the entrance to deeper relationships – the exact opposite of my previous understanding of conflict.

Repeated Conflicts

Several years ago, I was working in a school that changed administrators halfway through the school year. The new principal immediately implemented new programs that were familiar to her, but would require the rest of the staff to take time and energy to learn. I found myself getting more and more angry as I read the barrage of emails, and before I had a chance to meet her, I resolved not to participate in the new programs.

I had many thoughts running through my head. "She does not value my work. All she wants to do is make herself look good without acknowledging the expertise and systems already in place." The new principal's management style was a trigger for me, and with only some information, I went into 'attack' mode. The feeling of, "She does not value my work" is a recurring theme in many of my conflicts. It is one of my frequent spirals: I am not valued and I am not seen. As soon as something happens that brings this painful story to my attention, I attack. I react.

We all have triggers. We all have words or actions that get under our skin. They are well-worn stories stored inside our body, which is why they are so easy to revisit over and over again.

Conflicts inform you that something needs your attention. It is a signal that something in your world does not match your true self, and it requires you to take some action. It doesn't matter if the conflict resides within you, with a colleague, with your children, family members, the current political climate, or a complete stranger. Your conflicts are there to inform you that you need to think or do something differently.

When you take the time to think about all of the conflicts that you have, you will see a pattern. Your repeated conflicts lead to your crisis. Behind every crisis there is a story that needs healing.

You can pretend the story is not painful. You can act like the story does not belong to you, but this will not stop the conflict from returning and pointing you towards your crisis. Every conflict is a small crisis. It is like a helpless child asking for your attention. It is pointing to some story or some felt experience that needs to be addressed. If you can face your repeated conflicts, you can begin to transform yourself.

Rumblings of Your Crisis

Conflict is natural. Our entire universe has evolved as a result of problems or conflict that brought death and adaptation, and then resilience and life. Conflict is the foundation for growth. We have been practicing it for millions of years. The environment shifts, the earth gets colder or hotter, there is an elimination of a food source and there is a problem. As a species, our adaptation happened as a result of crisis usually around a depleting food source or a significant shift in our environment. We learned to adapt or we died.

Early humans moved out of their trees to brave the savannahs in East Africa. Moving into empty space meant exposure to danger, predators and the unknown. The brave ones were hungry enough to move across and find new food sources. Small groups formed into tribes that eventually worked together to accumulate resources. We know very little about how these early humans managed interpersonal conflicts. There is evidence that the old and the weak were pushed out of tribes and left to die. At some point, we know they cared for their sick and old. These small tribes eventually moved across the planet walking, eating and adapting to their environments. In his book *Sapiens* Yuval Harari suggests that our species began life very low on the competitive food chain. We only ate after the large animals, the small animals, the scavengers and the vultures had their fill. Curtis W. Marean, a professor at the School of Human Evolution and Social Change makes the case that humans have a genetic predisposition to cooperate with other humans that were not related to them. We are the only species that cooperate in groups larger than family groupings. Harari suggests that this cooperation was facilitated by creating common stories and beliefs. Harari writes, "…the truly unique feature of our language is not its ability to transmit information about men and lions. Rather, it's the ability to transmit information about things that do not exist at all. As far as we know, only Sapiens can talk about entire kinds of entities that they have never seen, touched or smelled. But fiction has enabled us not merely to imagine things, but to do so collectively." It wasn't until we began creating large-scale stories or beliefs that larger groups of humans began to cooperate. This allowed humans to dominate all the other species, despite the fact we were not the biggest, strongest or the fastest. Early hunter-gatherer communities worked both cooperatively and competitively. They managed conflict by giving power and leadership to dominant male members of the tribe, who probably used a combination of strength and capacity to lead. We have a biological history that managed conflict based on what position you held in your tribe. The more power and leadership you held, the more responsibility you carried and the more you got your way.

We still hold remnants of our early ancestors in both public and private organizations. The old traditional family model follows a pattern where men lead the household, women defer to their husbands, and children obey their parents. Traditional corporate organizations also manage conflict based on power and responsibility. These models value compliance. Although these practices of managing conflict based on power and responsibility are rapidly changing, it still holds true in both our public and private spheres. There are some advantages to this and this model certainly works when you need to take quick action, like getting everyone out of the house when there is a fire.

But our 200,000 years as humans and this tried and tested hierarchy has not given us much practice at expressing our point of view, or at managing difficult feelings and situations. Avoiding danger and searching for your next meal did not leave our ancestors with a great deal of time to practice listening and checking for understanding. The idea that we can talk about our conflicts and learn to understand each other's point of view to work and find solutions is new. It is only in the last sixty years that a growing number of families have practiced a co-parenting model where power is shared more equally, with both parents contributing financially, sharing household chores and parenting responsibilities. This sounds good in theory, but in practice, this has not gone smoothly. The evolution of sharing power within family members and communities at large, has taken place without the education, practice and encouragement our brains need to learn conflict resolution skills. Until very recently there was no specific curriculum that taught us, "How to get along."

We are wired to survive, not to thrive. As a result, our fear and insecurities can often rule the way we treat each other. For example, the person who brings in the biggest income often gets the better choice of family tasks. One parent can work to gain power over the other by manipulating relationships within the family. They can align some, or all of the children against the other parent, by undermining the other parent or inflating the value of their role in the family. Love, time and other resources can be used to ensure compliance and control.

Yet conflict still provides opportunities for communities to adapt, survive and thrive in changing environments. Conflicts, both personal and universal, require ecosystems to change. Ecosystems always favour balance, so systems tend to adapt towards a more equitable distribution of resources. This redistribution of power and resources can be hard for everyone. It takes practice and training to receive more power and it takes practice and training to have power and resources taken away.

Crisis Shows Up in Your Feelings That Hurt

The Feeling Brain

Your faithful companions in life's evolutionary journey are your feelings. The feeling brain is 100 million years old. Feelings are extremely important to our species. Our brain went to great lengths to carefully conserve feelings because they were critical for survival. When you avoid painful, uncomfortable feelings, you also avoid valuable information that needs your attention. Ignoring your uncomfortable feeling might feel like a solution, but it is only temporary. Eventually, it will work against you.

Anger

Anger energizes us. When we use that energy to actively do something, the anger is helpful and can give us the energy and courage to make a change. You can use anger to explode and pull a tantrum. This will temporarily relieve the tension by removing some of the stored energy, but if you don't address the root of your anger, you will just repeat this loop over and over again until you find the courage to heal the wound. If you hide, stifle, or pretend your anger is not there it can be dangerous to your body. The chemicals that are produced when you are angry are not meant to remain inside your body. When you avoid confronting your feelings of anger, those chemicals act on your body and over time create states of chronic disease, sickness, injury, depression, anxiousness or deep sadness. Anger is a feeling that is meant to help you move and provide you with energy to do something. From an evolutionary point of view, anger helped our species survive and adapt to changing environments. Think of anger as a signal. It's inviting you to acknowledge your responsibility and to take action.

It is there to help you attend to a story, a relationship or a circumstance that no longer belongs to you.

You will run into further complications when you try and use your anger to change the people around you. When you try and get everybody else to change so that you don't have to face your own wound, you may use your anger to avoid people from coming too close. You can use anger to avoid acting on and listening to the information that you are receiving. Anger can be dangerous when it explodes and gets passed on to something, or someone that is not what you are angry about in the first place.

I had a client in my energy medicine practice who was perpetually in conflict with his co-workers. As a result, he was constantly changing jobs. When he began a new job he would find a temporary break from his anger, but over time, he would once again find himself in conflict with a co-worker or his boss. After a few sessions, I wondered out loud, "Is it possible that you are creating or inviting this conflict, so that you can take care of some unfinished business?" When we went through the list of his difficult co-workers, we discovered some recurring themes: they were taking advantage of him, he was doing most of the work, they were not doing their 'fair share.' The feelings that repeatedly came up for my client all pointed to a story that hurt. Behind the anger, a deeper wound existed. When we examined his early stories, we discovered that many of his spirals stemmed from his childhood, where he experienced an unequal distribution of love and attention between his father and his other siblings. This childhood pain of not feeling loved helped to mould the story, "I do not deserve my fair share of love and attention." And since this childhood crisis had been stifled for so many years, anytime my client had the feeling of receiving less than his fair share, his old story would be triggered. Behind anger, there is often a well of deep grief.

Grief

Grief feels like the opposite of anger. Instead of feeling energized, you feel as if all of your energy has been sapped from the very core of your being. You feel as though all of your power has been stolen from you. Yet, grief and anger are two sides of the same coin. Just like anger, your body carefully conserves grief. Early humans survived by working as a strong collaborative unit. Sticking together helped early humans brave many challenges that came their way as they trekked around the world. The lives of tribe members needed to matter, as much, if not more, than their own. The by-product of all that care is grief. That is why, when a loved one or a relationship dies, it feels as though a part of your body has been cut off. In fact, electrically, that is exactly what is happening. Energy medicine works with energy fields that surround the body in several layers called auras. Auras respond to you and to your environment. We share electrical grid patterns with the ones we love, and when the relationship ends, the shared grid is severed. This split can contribute to intense physical, emotional and spiritual pain experienced by someone who is grieving.

Invite Them to The Table

So what can you do when anger, grief, hurt, or other painful feeling come your way? Feelings are meant to provoke action. They are there to propel you to do something. You stole my food and I need to do something about it. You are threatening my tribe and I need to do something about it. Feelings work best when we acknowledge them as soon as they happen. Confronting painful feelings is hard work. It takes a great deal of practice. One of the ways you get that practice is through face-to-face communication. When you connect with others, you receive direct feedback about who you are. You have your fears reflected back to you – your joy, shame, love and vulnerability. Face-to-face rehearsal teaches us to understand and identify our own feelings. That is why connecting with others is so important.

Give your full attention to all of your face-to-face encounters. It will take practice and at first it might not be easy, but you will get better at acknowledging your true feelings by staying present in your own experiences. Once you are aware of your feelings, you can address the information your feelings are trying to communicate. That might mean you need to move away from danger, or get some help so that you can decipher and unravel the messages your feelings are trying to tell you.

Your feeling brain evolved much earlier than your reasoning brain. Your feelings are smart and wise. They helped you survive. There is no good feeling or bad feeling - all feelings are information. You need to listen to the information your painful feelings are trying to tell you and take action. This is the way you adapt to your changing environment and eventually thrive.

Crisis Shows Up in Your Distractions and Addictions

Distractions

A distraction is any chemical, physical, mental or emotional activity that removes you from the responsibility of

managing a painful or uncomfortable experience. It is anything that takes you away from paying attention to a body
experience that is informing you that something needs to
change. A distraction is when you try to use sources outside of your own body's resources to feel good.

You can change your physical and emotional state
without using your body's natural resources in a number
of ways. You can do it by having a glass of wine, by taking prescription medication, by playing a game of Solitaire
on the computer, or by scanning your social media feeds.
Any of these distractions (and a million others) will move
you away from the responsibility of managing a painful or
uncomfortable felt experience.

There are times when distractions can help. If you are
completely overwhelmed and need a distraction, playing
a video game for example, can help you temporarily deal
with overwhelming stress. Eating a bowl of ice cream after
a big fight with a co-worker can temporarily help you manage your big feelings. However, playing a game or eating a
bowl of ice cream are short-term solutions that won't help
you get to the heart of the matter. The problem with distractions is that they are becoming the accepted currency
in our society for managing difficult feelings. If you constantly use distractions to manage your big uncomfortable feelings, you avoid dealing with the underlying felt
experiences. You avoid hearing the information and you
avoid unravelling and dismantling the old story. When
you practice your distractions often enough, they become
habits or addictions.

Some of the current cultural stories of 'happy' involve
having an abundance of money, fame, beauty, a 'happily
ever after' marriage with children and the white picket

fence, or one million viral video views. Yet any of these stories are only temporary distractions that take you away from staying in your felt experiences. Maybe the pain of parental rejection will be replaced once you have a significant other, or the trauma of being teased about a learning disability will no longer hurt once you are famous, or your ability to attract lots of sexual partners will replace the trauma of being teased about being a chubby adolescent.

Healing your crisis is an inside job. The success and positive rewards that you receive by using distractions as a crutch can temporarily help you avoid grief or trauma, but it cannot heal the wound. Your wound is inside of you and it will remain untouched by your distractions. It is up to you to uncover it and get to the source of your pain.

Addictions

Several years ago I was training for a half marathon and I developed Achilles tendonitis. I really wanted to race, and so my physiotherapist taped my foot. It was like a miracle, because suddenly, the pain was gone and I felt free to run. I completed the half marathon and I continued to tape my foot. Eventually, I ended up with a much more serious injury. The muscles and tendons that needed the practice were no longer being used, and rather than resting and allowing them to do the work when they were ready, I used tape to create a false sense of stabilisation.

That's what addictions do. They give you a false sense of stabilization. Dr. Gabor Mate, a physician who worked closely with people suffering from chemical addictions, describes addiction as, "Any behaviour where a person craves and finds temporary pleasure or relief in something,

but suffers negative consequences as a result of and is unable
to give up, despite those negative consequences." The reason
why addiction is a go-to for many of us is down to science.
Addictions give us relief from pain, or give us feelings of
pleasure because it is piggybacking on neural pathways
that already exist in our bodies. No drug works unless they
attach to a system that resembles the chemical equivalent
that works inside you. Endorphins are the body's natural
painkiller. When you are in crisis, or when you think you
are under threat or in real danger, your body releases endorphins to help you do what you need to do to get to safety,
or fight off a predator. Endorphins allowed you to manage
pain and survive. Our sexual organs, gut and immune systems carry many opiate receptors.

Gaba is an amino acid that acts as a neurotransmitter
in the central nervous system. It inhibits nerve transmis-
sion in the brain. It is the body's natural way of helping us
stay calm during stressful situations. When you chronically
use alcohol to regulate painful experiences, your body
decreases production of Gaba receptors. That is because
the alcohol is doing the work for them so they stop pro-
ducing it. This is your body's way of balancing itself.

Highly refined carbohydrates, heroin and morphine all
attach to a fixed opiate receptor that already exists in your
body. When you change the chemicals in your body using
an outside source, you are training your body to decrease
the chemicals that you produce to naturally help support
calm and wellbeing. When you use morphine or any of the
opiate prescription drugs, you are limiting your body's natural chemical pain relievers.

An addiction is a supercharged distraction. If you want
to move through your crisis, you will need practice using

your own body's resources to attend to the grief and the loss that exist inside the painful feeling. Any chronic distraction creates an artificial balance in your wellbeing. When you train your brain to continuously avoid painful felt experiences, you guarantee that you will repeat the crisis.

Crisis Shows Up in Your Root Exhaustion

I was a high school drama teacher for many years. Although I loved my job, there came a point in my life where I suddenly became overwhelmed with the work. I was making all kinds of mistakes, like filling in the wrong paper work for field trips and double-booking rehearsal spaces. I started losing my patience with the students. Lesson planning took twice as long and my ability to concentrate seemed to vanish. I did not understand what was happening to me. Eventually, I decided to take a few days off to try and get my bearings back. That first night, I decide to go to sleep at 8 p.m. "I'm not tired," I said to myself, "but I will get a fresh start on the next day."

The next day, I did not wake up until the afternoon. I had something to eat and then went back to bed. I did this for the next three days. I was exhausted and I did not even know it. It marked the beginning of a physical and emotional breakdown that required several months of recovery.

The tipping point came when I finally listened to my feelings of exhaustion in my physical body, but the truth is, my fatigue was everywhere – it was physical, mental, emotional and spiritual. Looking back, there were many clues that a crisis was brewing. I was single at the time and very lonely. I was watching friends and family get married and starting their families. I participated in all of their celebrations, ignoring my grief. I would go to a wedding and I was tired. I would go to a baptism and I was tired. I would help my friends with their babysitting and childcare, and although I loved being around their children, I would leave exhausted.

Look at your own life. There are thoughts that you have that make you tired. There are people in your circle that leave you drained of energy. Pay attention to what your body is trying to tell you, for these are all signals. Think about activities you do that bring you fatigue and defeat. Your weary bones are speaking to you. There is a theme in all of your root exhaustion, and left unchecked, it will bring you to your crisis.

An Opportunity for Full Scale Transformation

Coming into your painful radical interruption also contains a piece of magic. It provides you with an opportunity for full-scale transformation. Breaking free from a belief, a story, or an unhealthy relationship brings about space to create a new life. In fact, it demands this from you. There is a hole, or an empty space that cannot be put back together again. You get a chance to become your own alchemist, participating in a process that can transform the painful radical interruption into your personal gold. Suffering and brokenness can become the fuel to transform your life into strength, calm, and courage beyond understanding. Crisis is not just pain, brokenness and bad news. It also brings you a life with more freedom, confidence and purpose.

Recap

Crisis is a painful, radical interruption that causes you to stop living your life in your usual way. It is an opportunity for full-scale transformation. Although it feels sudden, it is a series of small, repeated cuts. These are hints that something needs your attention. Crisis begins with a single rip, another small rip and then another small rip - and then a thousand more. It is the Great Undo. It shows up in your repeated conflicts. It shows up in your repeated feelings that hurt, especially anger and grief. It shows up in your distractions and addictions. It shows up in your physical, mental and spiritual exhaustion.

What You Can Do

Below are several questions for you to answer that will help you to reflect on the material presented in this chapter. Depending on where you are in your crisis, you may want to explore these questions once you have tackled Chapter Two. Your death by a thousand cuts will take some time to unravel. Be kind to yourself. Take one question at a time and journal stories, thoughts and ideas that come your way. You may want to talk them through with a trusted loved one, or you may want to reflect on them by yourself, in quiet and solitude. You may simply want to write words or phrases that show up. You may also need to work with a counsellor, psychologist or support group. Make sure you reach out and get the help you need. As you work through the chapters you can come back and add more as you continue. This activity is not a race. It is a slow meander to help you reflect on all your parts – both the ones you love and celebrate as well as the ones you hate and hide.

My Repeated Conflicts:

- What was the last argument or discussion that you remember?

- What was it about?

- What were you feeling?

- How did it end?

- How do you feel about it now?

- What are the little things that annoy you?

- What are the qualities that you love about your mother? Father? Primary caregiver?

- What are the stories that you remember about these qualities?

- What are the qualities you hate about your mother? Father? Primary caregiver?

- What are the stories that you remember about these qualities?

- What are your repeated conflicts?

My Feelings that Hurt:

- What are the circumstances, habits or qualities that anger you most about others?

- What are the circumstances, habits or qualities that anger you most about yourself?

- List all the parts of your life that feel like unfinished business.

- Write about the first/last time you remember feeling deep sadness. What do these two stories have in common?

- Make a list of things you wish to complete, but have not yet done so. (Saving money to buy a car, reconnecting with a friend or family member, quitting your job).

- Know that grief, anger and sadness do not have to live in your body for your lifetime. You can take steps to move through and shift these feelings into healing and transformation.

My Distractions and Addictions:

- Keep a detailed log of all your activities for the next seven days. Include sleep, food, what you do at work, conversations, recreation activities, time on electronic devices, and feelings. Spend some quiet reflective time looking through the log.

- What are the strategies you use to manage your big feelings?

- What do you notice? What are your observations?

- What are the observations that make you happy?

- What observations bring you frustration, sadness or anger?

- How much time do you spend distracting yourself from difficult feelings?

- What steps could you take to change this pattern?

My Deep Exhaustion:

- What are the things that really tire you?

- Who are the people in your life that drain your energy whenever you spend time with them?

- What are the thoughts that tire you?

- What are the patterns in the thoughts, activities and people that drain your energy?

- What steps can you take to move away from the thoughts, activities and people that drain you?

Once you have worked through the questions, pay attention to the recurring themes. What are the patterns and thoughts, activities and actions that repeatedly show up? What can you do to take care of these repeated stories? Share the information with a trusted friend or a qualified counselor.

Chapter Two
You Are Crushed

*Unless we reach back through time and space to rescue
the stranded aspects of our child self and bring them
into resonance of the present where we provide them the
unconditional attention they require, we can't fully realize
peace.* **Michael Brown**

*Love your enemies because they are the instruments
of your destiny.* **Joseph Campbell**

There Is Never a Good Time to Die

MY NONNA HAD VERY big gnarly hands that were
full of knots and knobs and marks. They were anything
but smooth. Yet, those thick hands somehow managed

to manoeuvre tiny threads, knitting needles, yarns and stitches. It is not easy to make a well-fitted woollen sock, but Nonna's were little masterpieces. She tried to teach me how to repair the holes in socks. My attempts bore no resemblance to her expert repairs, for I did not put such heart into repairing my holes. Nonna is long gone, moved into fragments of in between space, swirling orbits of paradise lost and found, but my feet are still warm, surrounded by her stories.

Her hands bore both the shadow and light of a life lived sandwiched between world wars and poverty. Later, there was her depression, dementia and cancer – her slow, aching disintegration into nothing, which compressed all her unrefracted mirror bits into tiny black pieces of guilt, disappointment, fear and anger which eventually wove holes inside her body, painstakingly taking away all those memories where hope resided.

Unlike her knitted socks, Nonna did not manoeuvre the turns and corners in her own life so expertly. The edges of life terrified her. In fact, a lot of things about life scared Nonna. Just riding in a car scared her. I would gently tease her as she sat in the back of a vehicle, reciting the rosary in a concentrated whisper, unconvinced of the car's safety. Perhaps she had good reason, what with the manic driving and the narrow village roads that define all of Italy.

Somehow, the same hands that could meticulously pick the grass and weeds from the delicious baby radicchio, could not find a way to make the same delicate turns in her own life. How was it that the hands that could expertly manoeuvre the undos, turns, and circles of her stitches, fail to manage the undos and turns of her own emotional fabric? What is it that helps us to embrace all our undos? How do we turn and welcome all our holes made from moving inside our sacred circles?

You Are Crushed

When you are in the centre of your crisis, very little will feel familiar. And there is very little you can do, other than get your bearings. A painful, radical interruption means that your brain and entire body will be in some form of shock. You may have many thoughts, tasks and feelings flooding your body, but you will be unable to process this information.

The centre of your crisis is not the time to try and heal your childhood trauma, or mend a long-standing feud with your younger brother. It is also not the time to change your career or contemplate selling your house. Unless it pertains to the crisis, you should postpone any specific decisions about the past or the future. In the centre of your crisis, your brain is in survival mode, so you'll want to delay any major decisions until you have managed the present moment.

In the centre of your crisis your job is to survive. Your job is to deal with the present moment. Consider the fundamental questions: Are you safe? Are you breathing? Are you fed and hydrated? Have you moved your body? Have you spent time outdoors? Are you able to connect with people that you feel safe with? Can you name your feelings?

Are You Safe?

During my first year as a high school vice principal, a local resident called the school about a fight that was happening across the street. I quickly informed the school police officer and we both headed out towards the location of the fight. There was snow and ice on the roads and my expensive and very impractical boots could not manage the unpredictable landscape. I kept moving as quickly as I could. I suddenly realized that the six foot two police officer was *behind* me, walking slow and steady, even though he could have easily walked there in half the time that it was taking me.

He didn't say anything. He just looked at me like I was a little crazy. After we dealt with the situation, he turned to me and said, "Always walk into a volatile, unknown situation. You never run. You walk. That gives you time to spot any potential danger and it also gives time for everyone to see you coming. Half the time, the situation will disperse before you get there." This would have been great information to know before I ruined my boots, but I learned a valuable lesson – when facing a potentially dangerous situation, walk slowly and with purpose. It is a good practice when walking towards a fight and it turns out, it is good practice in the midst of crisis.

The first thing that you should do in a crisis is get yourself out of harm's way. Take that extra time to assess your situation and slow yourself down. It will help you to respond to your crisis. Your first task is to answer the question, "Am I safe?" Do this first. Time is your friend. You get yourself out of the burning building, you move to higher ground in the event of a flood, you get medical attention when you are involved in a car accident, you make sure you and your loved ones are safe when you shift away from an abusive relationship.

In the middle of crisis, everything either moves too fast, or completely shuts down. In both cases, your first task is to slow down, take care of your immediate needs and then assess the situation. Go slow. Move carefully. Get as much information as you can and walk with purpose.

Are You Breathing?

Overwhelm and shock will erode your brain's ability both to breathe and to reason. This is because your body will believe it is under threat. Since most of our evolutionary threats were physical ones, your body will favour a "fight or flight" response. This means that most of your body's resources will go to providing you with energy to do something physical. You don't need energy for digestion or fine motor skills or listening, so your body diverts energy away from these functions and gives it to the big muscles in charge of running away or making you strong in order to fight an oncoming predator. Whether you like it or not, when faced with a crisis you will tend to hold your breath, or breathe in very shallow, short breaths.

Take long slow breaths. Breathe in through your nose and focus on your belly expanding. Keep your shoulders still, away from your ears. This will prevent you from returning to your shallow breathing. When you take long slow breaths, you are disrupting the brain's arousal center. This is the part of the brain that informs the rest of the body that there is an emergency. When the arousal center is not activated, your body calms down.

Be still and breathe. This gives your body a chance to recharge your thinking brain. Once you are out of harm's way, get control of your breath. Big feelings will come at you in waves. Whenever the shock or feelings of being overwhelmed engulf you, your job is to help all the parts of your brain engage and participate in your crisis. The critical thinking part of your brain will come in handy as you navigate your crisis.

Are You Hydrated?

During a crisis, it is easy to forget the basic needs of your body, or to think that attending to these needs will not make a difference. Our bodies are 60% water. Every cell requires water to remove toxins and help bring nutrients into every cell. Water is vital in helping all the cells in your body carry out their functions and maintain equilibrium. When you are dehydrated, your cells shrink, including those in your brain. Dehydration contributes to feelings of confusion, irritability and feelings of overwhelm. If you are sick, in pain, or stressed, your body needs more water. In the centre of your crisis, drink water.

Are You Fed?

When you are in crisis, your body needs nourishment. The kind of food you put in your body impacts your thinking, feelings and physical wellbeing.

Our brains evolved as we walked and ate. We killed anything we could and then we ate it, often to extinction. We ate any vegetation that was edible, often to extinction. We would then move and adapt to a new environment and repeat the process again. Over time, our brains evolved and got bigger as we walked and increased our fat and protein consumption. Our brains are 65% fat and they grew the most when we went from a plant-based diet to an animal based diet. Up until recently, we ate fat, protein and very few carbs. Our bodies have not evolved to adapt to the amount of carbohydrates that our bodies are currently consuming. The bulk of the food that we see in the marketplace now is highly processed. Processed foods, especially sugar and refined carbohydrates, behave more like drugs that alter your gut and brain chemicals. They provide an instant hit of dopamine that temporarily provides you with a state of wellbeing.

There is a direct connection between the food you eat and the way that you feel. There is a symbiotic relationship between who you are, how you feel and the wellbeing of all the cells that coexist inside your body. You have more bacteria than you have cells in your body. The bacterium in your gut has a direct relationship with your brain, your feelings and your nervous system. For example, the chemical neurotransmitter, serotonin, which is responsible for balancing your mood, primarily lives in your gut.

Your body will take a beating in crisis. Your big feelings require good nutrition. The field of nutrition has many conflicting points of view around what we should eat, but there are several consistent guidelines that can help you make healthy food choices. In the centre of your crisis, nourish your body with the healthiest food you can. Slow down, prepare your meals and have loved ones help you prepare the food, if you can. Arrange to eat with others as often as possible. Slow down the whole meal process from preparation to clean up. What you eat and how you eat can make a difference in supporting your brain, your feelings and your whole being. Nourish your body so that it can support you in your crisis.

Have You Moved Your Body?

Early humans walked between three to seven miles a day. We still have bodies that favour movement, so, another way that you can help your body calibrate its equilibrium is simply by moving. Neurogenesis, (the growth of new brain cells), happens when you move. Intense bouts of high-energy movement will help you change your current mental state. It will be an important part of your recovery as you transform crisis into opportunity.

Move every day and make this part of your recovery. More importantly, make it a part of your life practice. It can be as simple as walking. It can be as diverse as ballroom dancing, table tennis, swimming, golfing, skateboarding or skiing. Find your passion. Do what you can. Then move every day. This is especially important if you are feeling depressed or sad, as movement increases the production of your body's natural feel good chemicals, serotonin and endorphin. Movement can help you energize your body. It is also critical when you are in a feeling state that has a tremendous amount of energy, like rage or intense frustration. Move so that you can release all of those chemicals that are coursing through your body. Movement will energize you when you don't have enough energy and it will calm your body when you have too much energy.

You brain works best when you are calm. In the centre of your crisis, take steps to move. For some of you, this is not going to be possible. If your crisis is a debilitating accident that has left you immobile or paralyzed, movement is tricky, to say the least. However, even if you *think* about moving your body, this will improve your feeling state.

Have You Spent Time Outdoors?

The Japanese practice of 'forest bathing' is the practice of spending time in forest environments. Studies found that simply hanging out in the presence of trees lowers your blood pressure, decreases cortisol levels, boosts your immune system and helps calm you down. This makes sense, given that the majority of our time as humans was spent outdoors in nature. Even if you do not have the luxury of living near a forest area, connecting with the natural environment will be beneficial. Garden spaces and urban parks are also good options.

Grounding is another technique that is beneficial to your health. Grounding is the premise that your body benefits when it is connected to the earth, sand and salt water. Our bodies come into contact with large amounts of positive electrons via Wi-Fi, cell phones and electromagnetic waves. To counteract all of these positive electrons, direct contact with the ground provides a negative grounding charge that neutralizes the positive electrons. Grounding reduces stress, inflammation, anxiety, muscle tension and chronic pain. It also improves sleep and speeds up the healing process.

Our bodies are designed to interact with the natural world. Spend time outside, preferably around nature. Even ten minutes a day spent connecting with nature will make a difference. If you are around trees, take a couple of good long deep breaths, as there is evidence that you will also get a bonus of forest bacteria that is good for your body. If you are lucky enough to live by water, especially ocean water, spend time near the shoreline. When possible, walk barefoot through grass, sand, water or dirt. Spending time outdoors is especially beneficial if you spend significant amounts of your day around electronic screens, or in confined, air conditioned cubicles.

Who Can Help You?

As a species, humans are designed to be around others. We survived by being in groups and it is hardwired into your DNA. If you are around people who care about you and if there is a sense of high regard and mutual respect, you feel better. Your serotonin increases, your ability to stay calm increases and the chemicals that support aggression decrease.

Human connection and being part of a thriving community are all related to longevity. Belonging to a healthy community is good for your physical and emotional health. It doesn't have to be your biological family. You can create your own communities and bonds. Being around others, helping others, taking care of members of your community, or even volunteering for the larger community helps you. Your brain works best when you are face-to-face, socializing, working, having fun and doing activities you enjoy.

You are not designed to go through crisis on your own. Quite often, your crisis will require you to get help, advice or support from outside your skill set. You are going to need the expertise of professionals, as well as the emotional support of loved ones. Once you are physically safe, you need to get informed. Allow yourself to be guided by people with specific skills. Crisis, addictions, family counsellors, emergency health caregivers, divorce or injury lawyers, bankruptcy trustees or credit counsellors, are all examples of professionals that you may need to consult in order to get more informed.

Can You Name Your Feeling?

Sometimes in my role as a school counsellor, I find myself working with a child who is experiencing great discomfort and they are unaware of it. "Suzy, your hands are curled in a fist and your eyebrows are meeting in the middle of your forehead. Your breathing is fast and it looks like you have all this energy in your body. I think you are having a big feeling!" When I voice my observations out loud, Suzy will inevitably acknowledge the discomfort and then together we can name the feeling and sort out what is happening.

Even though I have been working on feelings for a long time, I often find myself in the same boat – I am in great discomfort and I am unaware that I am having a big feeling. I have to remember, just like Suzy, to stop and check in with myself. What is my big feeling? The same goes for you. Take a moment to listen to your body. Acknowledge your feelings, without passing judgement. It will help you calm down. Explore what is happening in your body and connect with your felt experiences. If you have trouble putting the mixture of feelings into words, try talking to someone you trust, or try writing it down. Moving your body will also help you put words to feelings. The act of saying, "I am devastated" engages a part of your prefrontal cortex, the reasoning part of the brain, which then calms down the amygdala, the part of the brain that regulates your feelings. In other words, the act of becoming aware and acknowledging the feeling, lowers the intensity of the feeling.

Avoiding feelings that hurt, such as anger, shame, grief and fear will not change the fact that you are feeling them. Outwardly, you may deny any experience of these feelings, yet, inwardly, the limbic system, the part of your brain that alerts you to danger, is firing, informing your body you are having these feelings, and in some cases, increasing the intensity of the feelings. Pretending that you are not angry or afraid does not change the fact that you are angry or afraid. In fact, it may increase the intensity of the anger or fear.

Stifling your feelings can harm you. Even if you are acting like everything is okay, your body continues to release adrenaline, cortisol and endorphins. Your body thinks you are in immediate physical danger. All that cortisol and adrenaline trapped in your body need to be released. If these chemicals remain in your body, over time, they will harm you.

> # Recap
> The center of your crisis requires you to take care of your immediate needs. Your job is to make sure that you and your loved ones are safe and out of harm's way. Focus on your breathing, drink water, eat well and take care of your body by moving every day. Spend at least ten minutes of your day outside, preferably around nature. Find the people who can help you, and lean on the circle of people who you trust. Ask for and receive help from relevant professionals. Notice and name your feelings. Focus on your present concerns. Table any big decisions or concerns that do not have any immediate relevance to your crisis.

What You Can Do

Use the following questions to reflect on the material discussed in Chapter two. The questions below will help you to consider what you can do to get the support that you need. You can always come back to these questions later to reflect further on what safety looks like and feels like.

Are You Safe?

- What are the things that are within your ability to take care of you and your loved ones?

- Contact the appropriate emergency or support services immediately if it is necessary.

Are You Breathing?

- Begin your mornings and end your evenings with slow, focused breathing.

- Bring your hands to your belly and feel your belly expand as you breathe in and contract as you breathe out.

- When you can feel your thoughts spinning out of control, bring your focus back to your breath.

- Repeat this as often as you need.

Are You Hydrated?

- Drink water throughout the day, especially when you are feeling overwhelmed. Aim for eight glasses a day.

- If you are in shock, or feeling especially overwhelmed, take small sips of water.

Are You Fed?

- Eat simple, healthy foods.

- Try to eat your meals at a table and share the dining experience with others.

- Eat slowly and deliberately.

- Consume healthy fats such as avocado, olive and coconut oil, seeds and nuts.

- Take an interest in the ingredients of the food items that you purchase.

- Experiment with different vegetables at your farmer's market.

- Engage your family in the cooking process. Enlist the help and support of family and friends.

- Avoid all sugar and highly refined foods, including packaged breakfast cereals, potato chips or other snack foods, fruit bars or juices, all soft drinks including sugar free ones, as well as processed grains, especially wheat.

- Eating well is not about being perfect. Do the best that you can and acknowledge your efforts.

  Sample Breakfast: eggs and spinach, or nut butters on whole grain bread, or smoothies that contain fruit (apple, banana, berries), milk (almond, coconut, dairy), vegetables (kale, spinach, celery) and a healthy fat (avocado, nut butters, coconut oil).

  Sample Lunch: salad or grilled vegetables with a protein (chicken, fish, tofu or legumes).

  Sample Dinner: soup, roasted vegetables with a protein (dairy, meat, fish, or legumes).

Have You Moved Your Body?

Take at least 10 minutes to practice some form of deliberate movement. Some suggestions include:

- Take a walk outdoors, or go for a run.

- Do 50 jumping jacks, 20 sit-ups and 20 push-ups.

- Check YouTube for 10-minute high intensity work-out routines.

- Participate in sports or activities you enjoy. Swim, cycle, dance, participate in martial arts, or take a course that interests you.

- Always check with your doctor if you are starting a new activity, especially if you have existing health concerns. In fact, if you have not done so in the past year, get a full physical exam.

Who Can Help You?

- Seek out human touch and contact. Give and receive loving hugs, sensual and sexual contact. Book a massage if you are not able to receive loving touch.

- Enlist a trusted friend or family member and find out as much as you can about your crisis.

- Use the strengths of your community. Find out what supports you receive from any Employee Assistance Programs, Government, church or community supports. Do not be afraid to seek professional help.

Can You Name Your Feeling?

When you are feeling stuck, frozen or buzzing with a million ideas, there are some strategies that you can use to help you identify your current feeling state. Check to see how much energy you feel in your body. On a scale of 1 to 7, 1 meaning you have no feeling at all and 7 being over the top, what number would you give yourself? The amount of energy in your body provides you with clues towards the true feelings that you are experiencing. The chart below gives you examples of feelings connected to the amount of energy that you experience in your body.

Energy Level	Body Sensations	You are Feeling
1	No energy. Unable to move. Ears may feel like they are ringing. Very shallow breathing, no ability to concentrate. Eyes are sensitive to light. Unable to speak.	Petrified, Shocked, Frozen, Empty.
2	Low Energy. Shallow breathing. Slow movement. Hard to concentrate.	Depressed, Devastated, Wrath, Hopeless, Exhausted, Ashamed.
3	Tired, Lethargic, don't want to move or do anything.	Sad, Tired, Sleepy, Despair.
4	Able to think clearly and make decisions, even energy, able to think of the needs of others.	Calm, Even, Relaxed, Content.
5	More energy in the body, fidgeting, body feels uncomfortable.	Annoyed, Irate, Confused, Upset, Frustrated, Anxious, Worried, Unsettled.
6	Breathing is more rapid, you can feel your heart beating, increase in energy, racing thoughts.	Angry, Distressed, Afraid.
7	Hard to breathe, maximum energy in your body, limited ability to hold thoughts or listen.	Rage, Agony, Furious, Anguish, Outraged, Terrified.

Chapter Three
Unraveling the Story

You are not your past.

Tony Robbins

You are prepared by your past.

Joel Olsteen

You are your past.

Mamma

Mamma

I AM IN ITALY and I am fifteen years old. I am following my Nonna around her house, as she works. We are washing windows using vinegar, water, rags and muscles. I don't like the smell of the vinegar, but I notice that it is doing a nice job. We are talking and she is moving the bucket along and rinsing the rags. The water gets continually darker as she thoroughly cleans all the parts of the window. She shows me how to get to the corners and the edges. She doesn't speak too much, but I am asking her questions about our family. "What was your life like? How did you meet Nonno? What was my Mamma like when she was a little girl?"

She continues to move from window to window, and I continue to follow her as she answers my questions without pausing. She tells me that the men did not work on Sundays and that women took care of livestock, as well as the cooking and childcare on the, "Seventh day of rest". When she was first married to Nonno, he would help her with the chores on Sunday, only to be chastised by his brothers. So he stopped.

She continues to move and I continue to follow. We are in the kitchen now. "What do you remember about your Mamma dying?"

She has a dishrag in her hand and she is wiping near the sink. She puts the dishrag down. She moves towards me and sits down in one of the kitchen chairs. She holds my hands. Her well-worn, hard working hands still feel smooth and delicate. She talks in a reverent whisper, "When you are born, the first word that you say is *Mamma*. And when you die, the last word that you will say is *Mamma*."

She says the word Mamma with the same solemnity that I hear her use when I sit beside her in church. Nonna is closer to finishing her life than beginning it, but in her eyes, I see a girl who aches for the hands and the guidance of her mother.

Your First Home

Your mother is your first home. The first place where you define comfort, discomfort, need and satisfaction is a womb. You receive your first home and you stay there, in total darkness, in a space where you are powerless and at the complete mercy of your mother's choices. Your neighbours are incredible role models. Your mother's sacrum, her place of centre, lives directly below you. Right above you, her heart moves blood in and out, providing energy and resources throughout her entire body, receiving stories and giving stories, informing all of your body parts about the latest gossip and pertinent information about their neighbours.

For now, you are an integral part of the body itself. You respond to your mother's actions, her diet, her worry, restlessness, pain or unbound ecstasy. When she is happy, it sets off a chain of chemical experiences that change her physiology. Whatever happens to your mother also happens to you. When your mother feels threatened, she will have another set of chemical experiences: her body responds by sending out chemicals that will help her fight that stress. If your mother is stressed, if she is sad or angry, it will affect where her blood flows and what her body will see as a priority. This has an impact on your brain development. You begin life as a powerless receiver, unable to make decisions or communicate basic needs. In this protected space, you are in an environment that ideally delivers you with welcome, warmth and food. Regardless of quality, your 'Mamma Home' ultimately provides you with enough to live, develop and come out alive.

When you experience trauma in the form of a crisis or extreme pain, your body will instinctively return to the imprint of your first home. A major head trauma will put your body in a coma and you will retreat into the fetal position. When your spirit feels the stirrings of depression, when your body seeks deep rest, you return to the imprint of your first home. Your first home is so powerful, that even if your initial experiences are painful, dangerous and unhealthy, your body will still seek these same experiences. The womb is the place from which you measure all of your next experiences of home. You start with a set of stories and experiences that don't even belong to you.

Your First Six Years

The first six years of life are critical in shaping you. This is because your subconscious brain-training takes place at this time. From the time you are born, until the age of six, your primary brain state is theta waves – the same state as hypnosis. It is a time when you are an excellent receiver of information, but very poor at analysing it. This is an important evolutionary adaptation – it helped you learn information quickly and efficiently.

It means that all the information passed down to you is most likely the information that was passed down from your mother and father's parents, and their parents. The information that was passed on to you by your parents when they were under stress, experiencing trauma or feeling overwhelmed was imprinted on to you. There is a good chance that many of those old beliefs and values no longer work for you.

If a child feels like the relationship with the mother is at risk, this is traumatic. This information gets stored in the body. The same trauma response will then show up if a similar pattern gets triggered. You often do not even realize that you have triggered the trauma response.

Some research suggests that beliefs are passed down, at least in some part, through DNA. Beliefs can be embedded in your body via DNA - the part of the cell that records and creates blueprints for future cells. Your parents just don't pass down their blue eyes or lanky build. They also pass on their beliefs - both in how you are raised and through their DNA. Some of these beliefs are valuable and bring about positive, life-giving results. But others, especially those embedded in trauma and survival, tend to bring fear, disease and depletion.

These beliefs can go repeated and unchecked indefinitely. The way you react to hurtful and painful events stems back to your first stories. You collect these first stories and without even knowing it, they will define your future norms such as; how you should be treated, what counts as fair and equal, how you should use resources and plan for the future, how to be trustworthy as well as how to trust others. As you can see, a great deal happens before your sixth birthday!

You Are Not a Victim

At this point you might be thinking, "Oh great! All these trauma beliefs started before I was born. I was a child. This isn't fair!" Yet, right now, you are not too small to do anything. In fact you are ready right now to take the steps to start your journey. Your first job is to take 100% responsibility for where you are right now. You don't have to forgive everyone and everything that came before this moment, and it certainly doesn't mean that you must love your past. It doesn't mean that you are at fault for your past trauma, or that you are a bad person being punished, or that you deserved the terrible things that have happened to you. The pain, abuse, grief, trauma and unkindness happened. However, it does not have to run your present moment or control your future. Your current life situation is a result of everything you have received *and* everything that you have taught it. It means that you have the power right now to choose to move towards joy, rather than to move away from pain.

When you choose to move away from pain, your chief intention is to avoid getting hurt in any sort of way. Your whole being moves towards protecting yourself, hiding all of your important parts, your life-giving parts. Your energy looks inward. Your body is alert for any signals that danger is on its way. When you move away from pain, you send out signals to all of your systems, that danger is everywhere and you are not safe. It is an inward, protective process that moves you to see, feel and think about pain.

Victim thinking creates the perfect excuse for you to do nothing. It can be the reason you give yourself that it is dangerous to make a mistake. When you think that the world is out to get you and that you have to defend yourself from all those outside attacks, you lose out on all the opportunities to problem solve and work on your own solutions. You lose opportunities to train your brain to manage oncoming obstacles. Your brain needs many opportunities to fail and make mistakes. Unpredictability, stress and uncertainty strengthen your brain. It is how our brains learn resilience and perseverance. It is also how you increase your confidence in your ability to take care of your needs. In order to move towards a 'Culture of Thrive, you must take responsibility for your own feelings. When you sit and nurture the belief that your feelings are somebody else's responsibility, you lose the opportunity to heal. Uncertainty, mistakes, conflict, failure and crisis give you opportunities to break out of the rut.

For millions of years, your mistakes have been your greatest teachers. You may want to hide the bits that scare you, but it is important to own it all. Taking responsibility means you get to take control of your environment. Instead of looking for danger, you can choose to keep an eye out for possibilities and opportunities that bring you life.

Esther Perel's parents were Holocaust survivors who lived in a community in Antwerp, Belgium that was settled by 20,000 Holocaust survivors. Esther categorized two kinds of people in her Antwerp community – those who did not die, and those who came back to life. She describes community members, "Who did not die" as protective, always looking down, mistrustful and vigilant of their surroundings. Those who "Came back to life" looked up, always seeking a new adventure. They laughed and celebrated the present.

You can do something to take care of your current situation. When you move towards joy, your chief intention is to attract experiences that bring you life. Your whole being looks out for opportunities rather than pitfalls. When you move towards joy, you send out signals to all of your systems that joy is available to you and that you are willing to receive it. It is an outward, exposing process that moves you to see, feel and think about joy.

Trauma Beliefs

Your brain, for good reason, gives priority to trauma memories. This means your body learned to respond to life threatening situations quickly and efficiently. Getting lost in the supermarket could be a trauma memory that reminds you not to stray far from your mother and that may be important learning. It can also become a seed to the belief that you cannot take care of your own needs, or that it is dangerous to disobey. Through repetition, trauma memories can become trauma beliefs.

Some examples of trauma beliefs are:

- I am not enough.

- It is dangerous for me to tell the truth.

- My anger is dangerous.

- If I am seen, I am dangerous.

- My suffering is virtuous.

- My suffering keeps me close to God.

- I am the only person that I can rely on.

- I am unlovable.

- My feelings are dangerous.

- Wealth is evil.

- Good things don't come easy.

A small belief can create big pain and suffering. When you react with anger at a co-worker's comment about the quality of your work, it may be because this triggered your belief that you are not enough. When you curl under the blankets, frozen after someone has made fun of your body, this may trigger a story that you are not lovable. When you become aware of these triggers, when you acknowledge the root of your trauma beliefs, then you are more capable of responding to these triggers with a clear head.

Your First Story

Stories have a beginning, middle and an end. Fairy tales, fables and legends all describe journeys in a linear way in order to help the listener remember the important cultural lessons that are embedded in the story. They are also great devices for helping us remember and repeat the story. Linear stories are great for remembering and passing down information. The problem is, your life is not a fairy tale that can be lived in a straight line. You have a problem, you solve it and then you are happy. You are born, you live and then you die. Lines are only small segments of your life.

In the grand scheme of things, life happen as the universe happens – in large, sweeping, elliptical rounds with no real beginning, middle or end. From the tiniest "thing" that we can measure, to the largest "thing" we can imagine, life moves in a round. When you are living life in the part of the round that moves forward, you feel good, optimistic and expansive. It feels familiar and safe. When you live life in the part of the round that appears to move backwards, you can get discouraged, terrified, angry or uneasy. It feels like you are moving farther away from your goals, hopes and desires.

Crisis comes in the corners of the circle. It is the point of your life where you must make that left-hand turn and step out of the illusion that life always moves forward. Every time an unexpected struggle or disappointment enters your world, you are not sure if you are going to be OK. Every crisis, every 'left-hand turn' is a small death. It takes courage to face and recognize the left-hand turn, and you may even feel as though you are dying. In fact, this is exactly what is happening. You may have to make a few circles before you are ready to do anything about it, as you may not be ready to receive your death and transformation. Maybe you need to move inside the round, finding new tools or new friends that will somehow make 'the left-hand turn' more palatable.

You are going to do much better if you can learn from all of your stories without getting attached to your feelings of shame and disappointment. Look at all of your experiences as information - not good or evil. Own all your stories: the pleasant ones that make you feel proud, as well as the ones that make you feel small and insignificant. Your inherited stories make it very easy to pin the blame elsewhere for your problems. If only he would treat me with respect, or if only I could finish paying this debt off, if only I could lose 20 pounds, or when I get a divorce, or when I get over my cancer - then I will live my life! Blaming your inherited stories for your problems is a distraction. It is a way to avoid attending to your own inner work. An unresolved trauma belief can grow into something big and anonymous. As it grows, your life appears to get smaller and smaller. To move towards freedom, you must face the painful belief. You must make a conscious effort to choose to move past the loop of distraction and face your old belief. You sit still and you breathe.

This is when it gets tricky. When you challenge and dismantle an old story, you will learn both its truth and its lie. You may, in fact realize that you are NOT unlovable, and you may say, "Hey, I *am so* loveable! I am loveable just as I am, with all my opinions, failures and achievements, with all my conflicts and ecstasies, I am loveable!" You will rejoice and feel the initial freedom that comes from your body finally being unshackled from a burden that it was never meant to carry. *I am unlovable* is a myth! It is a lie! And this is a fact. Hooray!

But, you will also see the truth inside this old story, for indeed, you will come face-to-face with the fact that you are also unlovable. This truth will become evident when you begin to dismantle the old story. You will see the pieces about you that are unlovable. There will be many people, especially the ones you are most afraid of, who will gladly remind you of your unlovableness. You are *so* unlovable, they will say, with hurtful words or actions.

Your Healing is Dangerous

Your inner circle may not be ready to receive your new weightlessness. They may in fact feel terrified by it. Even though you may think that nothing about you has changed, that you still go to work at the same time, wear the same clothes, make the same kind of meals and so on, something has changed. Energetically, without any conscious aware-ness, the people around you know that something has shifted. They can sense your lightness, they can sense your new way of being. And they may not like it one single bit. Be prepared for a strong push back to your "normal" self by those that are close to you. You might notice that some people feel threatened by the new you and try to sabotage you. They may even try to push you back into the orbit that is your old story. You can count on losing some people around you. You may lose friends that have been faithful companions and steady supporters. You may find that your new way of thinking, even your new-found laughter and joy, bring anger, anxiety, or grief to the people around you. They will certainly try to stop you.

In my own life, I have noticed these points when I have taken a leap outside of my "normal". All my life I felt 'dumb'.

I struggled in school, especially in math, and compared to my twin sister, I did not excel academically. When I applied to graduate programs, I thought someone would discover my lack of intelligence and reject my application. When I was accepted into the program, I thought the school had inadvertently made a mistake and I had been the lucky recipient of their error. When I defended my PhD, I was terrified. I thought for sure, this was going to be when someone on the committee would recognize my stupidity and reject my thesis. I passed and although I was greatly relieved, I once again wondered if I had perhaps fooled the graduate committee. My insecurity was echoed back to me when one of my colleagues described the thesis as inferior. Despite the fact he had not read the thesis, I was crushed. I had to do the inner work of changing my old story. I could not rely on the outside world to validate my intelligence. I had to learn to acknowledge my own intelligence on my own terms.

The moment my move into school administration became public, some of my teacher friends began to exclude me from their circles. They would stop talking when I entered a room as if suddenly, I was no longer to be trusted. Some colleagues stopped inviting me to social events. It felt hurtful.

All these left-hand turns are dangerous work. You do not hold your old story alone. Your family, culture, religion, work and school spaces all hold old stories that contain trauma beliefs. In all of these old stories, you will discover your incompetence, your unlovableness, and your undesirability. Danaan Parry writes, "There is a Gandhi and there is a Hitler inside you and you embrace both, or you run the risk of projecting all of your dark side on the world and the people around you." There is much at stake at having you, "Go back to the way you were" but you cannot do that. You cannot go back.

When you are faced with your crisis, you have an opportunity to choose to move towards your new life, or stay in your old one that is dying. Hopefully, you choose door number one. Choose to live without the shackles of your old stories and trauma beliefs. Choose this small death, so that you can live your big life.

Fear is Easy

In every crisis, you have a choice. You can choose to confront the crisis, messy as it may be, or you can choose to avoid it, by staying in your loop of distraction and pretending that everything is OK. When you stick to your distractions you are setting yourself up for an even greater crisis. You can stick with what you know and choose to keep your old story. I have made that choice many times. Even though finding a life partner was something I truly desired, for most of my adult life, I believed that my life partner was something that would just come to me. All I had to do was be good, faithful and obedient and then, somebody would notice me. Yet, I was still single. One day a close friend challenged me, "Why aren't you working at finding a partner? If you put half the energy into finding a partner, that you have been putting in your career, you'd be married by now!" His words hurt but I knew he was right.

And so, I began facing my big fears. I put up a dating profile on several online dating sites and set aside time to "work" on meeting a partner. I went on a ton of dates. It wasn't easy. I took everything too personally. I painted every "no" as a failure and a sign of my unworthiness. Sometimes it was fun, but mostly it was difficult and scary. Eventually it got easier and after every encounter, I learned a little bit more about myself and how to date. It took me a very long time to break my old trauma belief.

One of the things that I learned along the way was that sitting in my pit of pitifulness had some real advantages. Believing that I was unworthy, or a failure gave me a good excuse not to face rejection. Believing that I had to be obedient and good in order to receive a relationship meant that I did not have to do the work of putting myself out in the world. I didn't have to expose my vulnerability or weaknesses. I could stay safe in the cocoon of 'I am not worthy' never exposing my terrifying story to those around me.

Your crisis is asking you to take stock of your life and to fix the parts that are broken, and more importantly, abandon the stories and beliefs that no longer serve you. The very fact that you are addressing your crisis means that you are growing. It means that you are acknowledging that your freedom and dreams are worth fighting for. Trust that a transformation will follow. A new life will follow.

Fear is easy. It lets you protect your vulnerability and your ugly. But it does not let you chase the desires of your heart. Your wants and wishes are on the other side of your fear. Challenging your fear will require effort, practice and a willingness to meet your vulnerability and weakness. The good news is that you have the capacity to make this happen.

Embracing Grief

So far you have acknowledged that you are not just a victim and that you are also responsible for your dark side.

Crisis requires you to leave behind the stories and beliefs that you thought were true, and in the process, feelings, beliefs and perceptions will be uncovered. Dogmas will be dismantled. That is a great deal of loss to take in.

When grief knocks at your door, it is your job is to receive it. No matter how unwelcome your guest is, it is a signal that the painful radical interruption is working its way through your life. Take the time to acknowledge the grief that shows up in your life. Don't smother it, or shove it under the carpet. Work through it. Buried grief will always return. While embracing this period of grief, do what you can to take care of you. Don't forget to breathe. Make sure you are fed and hydrated. Move your body, connect with the outside world and loved ones, and be kind to yourself. Grief can sap the life force from your bones, making you feel lethargic. Everything may feel like a great effort. Try thinking of grief as a guest and with that in mind, be careful not to throw your guest out too quickly. Work through your grief slowly, in your own time and remember that grief has a different timeline for everyone.

When your energy begins returning and you feel ready to enter the stream of daily life, this will be your cue to begin sending your grief on its way. Not that grief will always leave. The death of a child leaves an imprint that will forever shadow a parent. No matter how traumatic your crisis has been, there will come a time when grief no longer holds the choking grip around your chest, but instead, finds a space where both joy and sorrow can live side by side. Eventually, your crisis will become the compost that nourishes your new story, your new life. Surviving your crisis will give you the strength, courage and the wisdom to let go of the feelings that no longer belong to you. It is not simple, easy or quick, because crisis and transformation require hard work.

You look at your undos and trust that going backwards to retrieve some of your painful stories will somehow provide you with the key to your well-being. You do this one small courageous step at a time.

You Have to Die

Crisis invites you to make choices and decisions that you never thought were available to you. You realize that now is the right time to leave your broken marriage, to say no to your children, to quit your job, file for bankruptcy, or own up to your learning. Any one of these choices require you to give something up and that something is often attached to a story you believed would be with you for the rest of your life.

There is no getting around this part. You have to die. Living life in a circle and making a left-hand turn means that you abandon the familiar, and experience some form of dying. It means that now is the time for you to let go of the idea that you would never be divorced. It means you let go of the idea that you are the perfect parent, or at least a better parent than your own parents. You let go of the idea that you will always be healthy, or that the values and beliefs you grew up with are right. Crisis will break some piece of you and it will hurt.

The pain might feel so intense that you may be tempted to escape it. But taking the loop of distraction will only delay the suffering, and every time you avoid your pain, you create more of it. After your binge, your hangover, your momentary escape, you will once again open your eyes and your suffering will greet you. Receive your crisis, your loss, disappointment and shame. Your unwelcomed guests will not stay forever, although they will leave you with some reminder of their visit.

You may find that this pain, this death, is so difficult, that you will be tempted to quit. Keep going. Your life is not over. Stay present in your pain, remembering to do everything you can to take care of your needs. Are you breathing? Are you safe? Are you fed and hydrated? Have you moved your body? Who can help you? You are still here, alive - and you will move past this pain.

To live well is to practice dying thousands and thousands of times. A good life is about receiving repeated opportunities to practice dying. Acknowledging the painful aspects of life means that you are willing to engage in the pain, with the understanding that an old story is dying. By accepting it, you are allowing the pain to guide you towards a new story.

So, you die a small death, or a very big one. You dismantle your old story. This is practice for your final death, your final transformation where you leave your body and begin a new life inside another form. As life is always full of paradoxes – The more you handle grief well, the more you can move through conflict well, the more you get comfortable with dying, the better you become at living. It brings you the strength and the resilience to live in the now. That is what embracing crisis is all about. Crisis helps you to live well and to have the courage to receive contentment. You enter grief, suffering and conflict with the confidence that transformation will meet you at the other side. You are alive and you are learning to recognize and embrace your final dying.

You want to move through your crisis and come back to life. You walk towards your pain, this death that stares at you, and you dance together for a while. And then you survive, until you have the resources to thrive. You choose not to relive your crisis; instead, you take your second chance and you savour every minute of it. You keep your head up and you look for ways to seek more life.

Recap

Your first home was your mother's body. You began this life in a receiving state, powerless to do anything about what you were receiving. Your first stories of receiving define how you view your world today, and are largely established by the time you are six years old. Since evolution favours trauma memories as a way of surviving, you store and remember those memories and beliefs first. Many of these trauma beliefs are toxic and unhealthy. You have the power to change that viewpoint because, today, you are taking 100% responsibility for where you are right now. You are not a victim. You can choose to stay where you are with your trauma beliefs, if you like, or you can choose to summon all your strength, courage and wisdom and allow those old trauma beliefs to die. You allow time and space for grief. You enter your suffering but do not hang out there for too long for you choose to come back to life.

What You Can Do

Your crisis holds many clues as to the nature of the trauma belief that is inviting its death. They will come to you in the form of feelings and stories. The best way to pry them out and understand them a bit better is by writing, reflecting and getting support from loved ones. Below are some questions to help you to discover your trauma beliefs. Reflect on your responses through a journal. Share your responses with a trusted counsellor, support group, family or friend.

Your Parents

- What five words would you use to describe your biological mother/father?

- What do you consider her/his weaknesses? Strengths?

- What is your favourite memory of your mother/father? Least favourite?

- What do you appreciate most about your mother/father? Least?

- What was your mother's role in your household? Father's role?

- What is your mother/father's super power? Her/his kryptonite?

- How would you describe your relationship with your mother/father today? When you were six years old? When you moved out? Graduated? Introduced your first partner? Married or moved in with a significant relationship? Other significant events?

Significant Relationships

- What are five words you would use to describe your partner?

- What do you consider her/his weaknesses? Strengths?

- How did you meet?
- What did you notice first?
- What was most attractive about your partner?
- What do you appreciate most? Least?
- What do you remember about your first disappointment?
- In what ways does your partner remind you of your mother or father?
- What is their super power? Kryptonite?

Your Turn

- What are five words you would use to describe yourself?
- What do you consider to be your strengths? Weaknesses?
- What is your best memory? Worst memory?
- What do you appreciate most about yourself? Least?
- What parts of your life do you feel you have no control over?
- What is your super power? Kryptonite?
- What parts of your story can you take charge of today?
- What is one fear you are willing to tackle today?
- Who can help you?
- What steps can you take to challenge that fear.

Revisit Your Own Stories

Take the time to reflect back on some of the old stories you wrote about in Chapter One. What other information can you add to your reflections? What are the repeated themes that continue to show up in your conflicts?

- I am not enough.

- It is dangerous for me to tell the truth.

- My anger is dangerous.

- If I am seen, I am dangerous.

- My suffering is virtuous.

- My suffering keeps me close to God.

- I am the only person that I can rely on.

- I am unlovable.

- My feelings are dangerous.

- Wealth is evil.

- Good things don't come easy.

Get Help from the Experts

Remember that some of this work will require the expertise and support of professionals and it will be important that you get that help. This will especially be true if you are struggling to untangle from significant distraction or addictive behaviours.

Chapter Four
Opportunity

During the bombing raids of World War II, thousands of children were orphaned and left to starve. The fortunate ones were rescued and placed in refugee camps where they received food and good care. But many of these children who had lost so much could not sleep at night. They feared waking up to find themselves once again homeless and without food. Nothing seemed to reassure them. Finally, someone hit upon the idea of giving each child a piece of bread to hold at bedtime. Holding their bread, these children could finally sleep in peace. All through the night the bread reminded them, "Today I ate and I will eat again tomorrow."

Dennis, Sheila and Matthew Linn

But maybe the death you fear is not simply the death at the end of your present life. Maybe the death at the end of your life won't be so fearful if you can die well now.

Henri Nouwen

First You Cry

I AM ON MY way to my mom's house for the afternoon, where we are going to make antipasto. I am not having a good day. I am trying to keep my rising stream of grief and disappointment under control, but I am not doing a great job. I am 45 years old, but I feel like I am seven. Two obsessions that have been my constant companions have come to a head. For my whole life, my spirituality has been intertwined with the Catholic Church. Daily mass, a desire to become a missionary, a disastrous stint as a volunteer, a fascination with liberation theology had slowly evolved into disillusionment and a realization that my core beliefs had quietly moved farther away from the church's core principles. I was slowly hanging on with a smaller and smaller grasp, yet I was unwilling to leave my childhood spiritual home.

My second preoccupation was my long search for my life partner. After years of dating, I was engaged and planning to marry. Although the church did not recognize my partner's first marriage, he was expected to complete the same annulment procedure as if they had recognized the marriage. This was the final rule I could not swallow. So, I resign myself to hosting my wedding outside the Catholic church. I am devastated.

I drive to mom's house, to help her make antipasto. In an Italian home, the celebration of food is a spiritual practice. It is early morning and my mom is still in her nightgown, but the kitchen is already organized for the event. The jars are sterilized and cleaned. The piles of vegetables are ready. My inability to hide my feelings means that by the time I've taken my coat off, I am bawling my eyes out. I see my restless mom trying to figure out what she needs to do or say to make my tears subside, but they just keep coming. Finally, she sits down, one eyeball on the piles of vegetables, jars and supplies, torn between making antipasto and her daughter's tears.

"All right," she says, "first you cry, and *then* we make the antipasto."

The Itchy Wound

By now, you have worked through some of the "What You Can Do" strategies found at the end of Chapters 1, 2 and 3. You have taken care of your immediate needs. You have taken steps to unpack some old beliefs that no longer serve you. You have started some routines that are beginning to form habits and you are getting the support and information you need to work through your crisis. You have met with grief and you have acknowledged your losses. You have cried and now it is time to make the antipasto.

You haven't noticed, but things in your life have already started to change. When you hear yourself saying, "I am so tired of living life in this small box, I want more," it is a signal of progress. Right now, you might be feeling impatient to see some big changes – you want more of something, even if you are not sure what that is. Your restlessness is a sign of progress. You are in the uncomfortable place where your wound is healing, laying down new skin, new cells, new tissue. Your skin is itchy and uncomfortable. It is tempting to pull off the protective scab but it is not quite time yet.

You have already taken many steps in your thousand-mile journey, and your desire to want more from your life signals more of your healing. Instead of looking to just get through the day, you have moved your gaze towards what will happen next. Instead of surviving, you have moved your attention to thriving. Small imperceptible changes, repeated over time, will bring you the life you desire.

This chapter will provide a number of strategies for you to practice. There will be several tactics that you can use to train your brain to acclimatize to a new story. These approaches will be your bread. Every time you complete these tasks, they will be a reminder that today you choose to die to your old story and begin your new one. You have created an opening, an in between space, that allows for the dismantling of an old story and the radical space for a new story to emerge.

It begins as soon as you become aware that you would like to *feel* differently. Maybe your old tribal belief, "To be seen is dangerous" feels constrictive, suffocating and you don't want to feel that anymore. When you become aware that you want a better feeling, the new story becomes available to you. Your discomfort signals progress. You are alive, and today, you choose your big life.

From Survive to Thrive

Evolution has wired our brains and bodies for survival. Our first impulse, our memories and our chemical make up are all designed to survive our environment and living conditions 30,000 years ago. We were still hunter-gatherers and just starting to experiment with farming and domesticating animals. Our threats were immediate – food, shelter, physical attacks from other tribes, human species, animals, the weather and the land. We still spent the bulk of our time outdoors, in small groups, working on our day-to-day physical needs. This has little resemblance to our modern day existence.

Survival skills are not the same skills required to thrive. In fact, they are often the opposite impulses. In order to move towards thrive, you need a new set of skills and awareness. You will have to learn to become aware of your first impulse, your survival impulse and do the opposite! You are going to need to learn to engage the parts of your brain that are NOT designed to react to physical threat. Instead we practice working with the pre-frontal cortex, the reasoning part of the brain that is slower, but makes decisions based in the present moment but it also allows you to consider your future self. Your reasoning brain will help you make choices that favour the all-important long view. Your new stories are going to require brain training that favours the parts of your brain that look beyond the present moment, beyond immediate danger and beyond physical threats.

Disruption

What are the strategies that help you move towards the new story? Remember, brains love practice, repetition and behaviour. In order to make the new story 'stick' you follow it up with repeated behaviour. Your thoughts work best attached to action - and this is where disruptions come in.

A disruption is when you use your body's resources to manage feelings that hurt. It is the opposite of a distraction. A *distraction* is any chemical, physical, mental or emotional activity that removes you from the responsibility of managing a painful or uncomfortable experience. A disruption

works *with* your body to help you stick to the felt experience and maybe take the edge off some of the intensity. It
uses your brain's natural reward system to solve problems,
manage feelings and address the information that comes
with big feelings. Disruptions are conscious practices and
behaviours that train your brain to move you towards joy.
They are the small repeated habits that over time, provide
you with the skills to feel better and to live a better life.

There is nothing fancy about disruptions. They are
brain hacks, continuously repeated until they become
unconscious habits. They are simple practices that may be
difficult initially, but over time, become effortless. Like a
good video game, they are easy to learn and hard to mas-
ter. Yet, they are the key to transforming your crisis into
an opportunity. Read through the disruptions below. Take
your time and think carefully about each of the disruptions
without deciding which ones you will try and which ones
you will table for another time. Disruption examples will
be examined in more detail in the next two chapters.

Distractions Versus Disruptions

Distractions	Disruptions
Video games, social media, apps.	Hang out with people who care about you.
Highly refined foods, sugar, simple carbohydrates.	Move, walk, jog, spend time outdoors or in nature.
Blaming someone else for your big feelings.	Heavy labour, weight lifting, High intensity workouts.
Expecting someone else to fix your discomfort.	Meditations, stillness, breath work.

Distractions	Disruptions
Hurting yourself.	Make a decision and follow through with it.
Drugs and alcohol.	Taking responsibility for your feelings and managing your own discomfort.
Self pity/Negative self talk.	Name the better feeling story.

A Disruption Can Become a Distraction

Not to get too complicated, but I should mention that disruptions can easily become distractions. Whenever you use your body's natural resources to *avoid* feelings that hurt, you are using a disruption to distract you from doing the difficult work of taking care of your feelings. You can form an addiction to working out. You can become a workaholic to avoid working on your marriage. You can meditate or pray intensely in order to avoid dealing with your depression and the underlying pain beneath it. There are an infinite number of creative ways you can avoid taking care of your feelings that hurt. It will be tempting to "go back to your normal" once you have recovered from your crisis but you have come too far to settle. Minimize distractions. Continue to explore and practice disruptions.

Focus on the Better Feeling Story

Our thoughts produce a physiological experience. Our thoughts can change our internal physical landscape in a way that can help you or harm you. Your self-talk can empower you to make a change to feel better, or it can suppress your ability to make that change. You can hurt someone with unkind words. The same is true when you say these words to yourself. If early on in your life, you were made to believe that you were bad, unworthy, ugly, lazy or dumb, over time these words become your beliefs. These beliefs get stored in your body. Any belief or story that does not align with your true nature is toxic. You may have spent a lifetime nurturing these toxic stories but they do not have to be your future.

Developmental Biologist, Bruce Lipton suggests that the function of the mind is to create consistency with your beliefs. When you focus your thoughts on your strengths and possibilities, you are increasing the opportunities for your body to be calm and focused. Calm and happy bodies release dopamine which increase pleasure and motivation, while decreasing anxiousness. Calm bodies release serotonin which increases pleasure and decreases aggression.

Redirect your thoughts and words towards the better feeling story. Support your wellbeing by using language and words that elevate, challenge and support your thoughts. Use words that help you focus on where you want to go, instead of focusing on where you are afraid to be. The words that you tell yourself need to move you in the direction of your heart's desire. If you keep using harmful words, you'll deplete your body of the resources it needs to help you take care of yourself. It discourages you from practicing habits that move you towards success.

More Than Words

Words and thoughts are powerful, but they are not the whole story. You can say, "I am skinny", but if you continue eating unhealthy food and leading a sedentary life, no amount of positive thinking will help you to lose an ounce of weight. You can say, "I have one million dollars in the bank", but if you don't put in the hard work that is required, words and thoughts will not increase your bank balance. Your thoughts are like the yeast in bread: you can't have bread without it, but you need more ingredients and effort in order to make it happen.

Find ways to disconnect from the story you are currently stuck in, the one you have repeatedly told yourself and those around you. This requires you to tell a new story about who you are. I am working towards being a firm and kind mom. I am able to save my money and manage my financial health. I have the ability and willingness to find a job that values my passion, energy and enthusiasm. I have the capacity and courage to attract a healthy, smart, loving life partner.

You now have the opportunity to practice skills and habits that will support your healing. These opportunities come in small moments. For example, if you catch yourself in the middle of a tense argument, instead of reacting in an explosive damaging manner, take a breath and pause. You can re-write your usual negative self-talk or reactions. You can remind yourself that you are strong and able to make a change. It is time to move your gaze towards where you want to be. Instead of looking back and feeling awful about how you handled a situation, use your discipline to look forward, towards the life you want to lead.

Creating habits take time. You are not always going to catch yourself in the middle of an argument or use your disruption strategies to manage your big feelings. You will make mistakes. Remember, conflicts and mistakes are a part of being alive. It is about working on what you say to yourself after the mistake or the conflict that counts. If you can think about the story in a way that supports growth, then you have turned it into a learning situation. You can go back to your loved one and say, "Hey, I don't think I handled last night's discussion well. I want to try and find a way to do this so that we both get a chance to listen to each other's point of view. Can we try again?"

As soon as you focus on what can be better, your body will be in a learning state. You don't want to get used to the feelings and the chemicals that support your sense of helplessness. Once you have experienced the disappointment or shame, you don't have to stay in it. You can turn that around and practice the discipline of moving towards where you want to go.

It Takes Time

You are not trying to make it better all at once. That's what an addiction does. I'm going to get drunk and forget about this pain. I'm going to gamble and I'm going to forget about how hurt I feel. I am going to play a video game and I'm going to forget about my failure.

Choosing the better feeling story is about doing one small practice at a time to move you towards your healing. When you keep saying, "My life is horrible", then all you're going to see is your horrible life. Change the story and then do something that reinforces the thinking. For example, you can implement small, but consistent steps to develop a stronger bond with your children. You can take small, repeated steps that will move you towards a healthy lifestyle. The more you practice reframing your story, the quicker you will move towards success.

Developing Resilience

Resilience is the ability to manage stress, change and uncertainty. A study from Norman Garmezy, a developmental psychologist and clinician at the University of Minnesota, found that high levels of resilience did not correspond to the subject's level of trauma, or their socioeconomic status. It all came down to outlook and perspective. Individuals with strong resilience skills were the people who could frame their challenges and crisis as opportunities for growth, learning and success. In other words, people who practiced positive self-talk were better able to manage their stress levels. By contrast, people who framed their problems as a catastrophe, or the fault of someone else, or unsolvable, did not develop strong resilience skills.

What you tell yourself about what is happening to you determines how you handle the problem. What you say to yourself about your challenges either trains your brain to cope, or trains your brain to shut down and feel powerless.

Let's just say you yelled at your children and sent them to their room for acting out and having a meltdown in the supermarket. You are overwhelmed, tired and embarrassed - and maybe you are feeling guilty. You might be thinking, "Why did I yell at them? Why didn't I just leave the store and tell them to stop? I am a terrible mother! I promised myself I would never do the things my mom did to me and here I am, doing the same thing. Why can't my kids just respect me and appreciate me more?" The story you tell yourself produces chemicals in your body that shut down your ability to think of solutions.

After you have calmed down, you can take the time to reflect on the incident. Maybe you will acknowledge that, "I didn't like the way this felt. I want to do this differently.

I have the skills and the courage to make better decisions. What can I do to change this scenario for the next time? What can I do, right now, to feel better?" The answer to that question is going to look different for everyone. Maybe it means making a phone call to someone who can help you come up with solutions. Maybe it means taking the time to find new strategies to cope with situations like this. Perhaps it means you need to acknowledge that it's important to take care of your own needs more, so that when conflict shows up, you will feel better prepared to cope.

Pay Attention to Your Lonely

Being on the outs with your tribe could cost you your life. It is no wonder we do what we can to avoid feeling lonely. Our cells have millions of years of practice equating lonely with death. Feeling lonely can be painful. It is the experience of feeling discontent or sad at the lack of human connection. It has nothing to do with the number of people who surround you. Quite often, feelings of loneliness arise as a product of your circumstances. If you are living a good life, lonely is normal. People you love die. People you love hurt you. You feel misunderstood. You are in a community or situation where you feel out of place. You don't see your reflection in the people around you.

It is important to remember that feeling lonely is a temporary state. It will move with you through the ebbs and flows of life. There will be times when your life will be full of connection and human contact. There will be times when the flow of community will be easy and effortless. And there will be times when it will be work and full of effort, often at times when you don't have the energy, or resources available to you. Some of my greatest moments of loneliness have been the hours I spent in a darkened room, unable to move without excruciating pain, during my years struggling with undiagnosed fibromyalgia.

Feeling lonely can also be a sign of transformation. In my energy medicine practice, when a client expresses feelings of deep and painful loneliness, it can be a signal of an impending transformation. That deep sense of disconnect with the outside world may be the early signs of your awareness that something needs to change. Something big. Maybe you realize a family 'norm' is no longer okay with you. Or you have evolved out of your tribe. Or the balance of power in your marriage needs rearranging. Or the way you have taught your children to treat you now needs an overhaul. Maybe you now realize you have been spending money on stuff in order to cover up your feelings of, "Not good enough."

Loneliness can be a powerful sign that transformation wants to push its way forward. Don't be too quick to judge your loneliness as a sign that your life is crappy, or that you lack community. There is much more to your lonely. You might be in the throes of a healing, a rebirth and a bigger life.

Routines and Repetition

When I was a teenager, I used to bake these plain, coffee-dunking cookies that my dad ate for breakfast. I baked them so often that I stopped looking at the recipe. Inevitably, there was the occasional mishap - like the time I forgot to put in the baking soda (the offending hockey pucks were fed to the family dog), but mostly, the cookies landed on the family breakfast table. I can still remember some of the ingredients: 6 eggs, 1 1/2 cups of oil, 2 cups of sugar, the zest of one lemon. For some reason, the amount of baking soda escapes me.

There was something comforting and calming about repeating the same recipe. I liked the predictability. I liked knowing that they were being put to some practical use. Repeated behaviour is one of the most powerful learning strategies. Every effort you make to create small, repeated behaviours that move you towards your passions and desires is success. In terms of learning, what you do repeatedly wins. What are the routines that you can begin that will have an impact on your success?

Single Focused Time

Our brains were not designed to multi task. In fact, they don't. Brains task switch. You participate in one mental activity and switch to another activity. When you participate in task switching, it takes more time to complete a task, you make more mistakes and you are less productive. Single focused time is the most efficient way for your brain to complete a task. Eliminate distractions. Our brains works best when you can devote single focused time to the task. Set aside time and energy to work on your goals.

If you want to complete a task or challenge, set a specific goal. Set a specified time, with a written set of actions and schedule blocks of time that you devote to your goal with no other tasks or distractions.

Finish Tasks to the End

Twenty years ago, an experienced runner mentored me through my first half marathon. During our training runs, she would give me advice on appropriate running gear, how to breathe, hold my body and when to refuel. She also taught me how to end the race, "When you get to the last 400 metres, stop, tuck your shirt in, adjust your hair, your hat, and make sure your number is well displayed. There is going to be a photographer at the end, and you want to make sure you look good for the picture." At the time, this felt like a gross waste of time and energy. Who cares about looking good for the finish line? I just want to get across it in one piece! For my mentor, the end of the race was not just the finish line, it was ensuring that the record of my ending put me in the best possible light. The finisher's photo, and a good finisher's photo was more important than finishing a few seconds earlier.

Extending the definition of finishing helps build excellence and patience. A job is completed when everything is finished past the task. The car is washed, after all of the garbage and cleaning products are put away in their proper place. The homework is truly completed once it has been reviewed, checked and put away in its proper place. The laundry is completed after it has been taken out of the dryer, folded and put away. The project is completed once it has been reviewed, evaluated, and set up for future success.

Finishing is important for your brain. It helps you push past the points of, "I can't do this." It stretches your ability to take risks and problem solve. It builds grit, resolve and accountability. Tuck your shirt in, adjust your hat and make a plan to finish. There might not be a photo for you at the finish line, but your increased confidence, resilience and patience will be your medal.

Make a Decision

Several years ago, I was struggling in my role as a Vice Principal. I was having a hard time figuring out what I could do to change my situation. For over a year, I made several attempts to make my job "fit" my passions. I tried to organize a curriculum that focused on sustainable trades and carbon free living. I applied for jobs that were closer to where I lived, to minimize the long travel times that added to my long working hours. I tried to streamline the tasks I hated. I tried collaborating with colleagues that I liked and who brought me energy and joy.

All of these decisions were not the 'best' decision, but eventually they led me to the right decision. I was able to step down from my role, and take a position as a counsellor, a job that was more aligned with my beliefs and my skill set. In your own life, there will be times when you feel stuck and unable to decide what to do next. Remember that moving forward does not have to always be the "perfect" decision, in fact sometimes it just has to be a choice that will help you get unstuck. When you make a decision, and follow through with it, you will help your brain open up to more possibilities and opportunities.

Invite Uncertainty

Studies found that seniors walking on cobblestones rather than smooth paved roads increased neural activity and learning. Resilience is all about stretching the brain just outside the comfort zone and pushing beyond what you know. We need uncertainty to develop and evolve. Challenges are good learning opportunities wrapped in discomfort, pain and stress. You need a little pain and suffering to learn. Optimal environments are the equivalent of smooth pavement - and you don't want that.

Safe environments guarantee that you will *not* get the practice you need to develop a resilient brain. Thriving requires repeated practice inhabiting uncertain, unpredictable spaces. Every time you problem solve, or manage your discomfort or stress, you are managing uncertainty. You are training your brain to thrive.

Recap

When you begin to feel restless and frustrated with your current situation you are already healing. You are training your brain to create a new story. You do this through repeated disruptions. A disruption is any behaviour that works with your body to manage feelings that hurt, by using your body's natural reward system to solve problems and address the information that comes with big feelings. Examples of disruptions include; Using positive, solution based self talk, practicing perseverance and resilience skills, making a decision, inviting uncertainty, creating consistent routines, completing tasks to the end, setting specific goals, and allowing space for loneliness to inform you about what needs to change in your life.

What You Can Do

Pay Attention to Your Lonely

- What are the activities that you do to distract yourself from feeling lonely?

- Write down your earliest memory of feeling lonely. How old were you? What were you wearing? Where were you? Do you remember what was happening before that moment? How did you handle the feeling?

- Write down the last time you remember feeling lonely. Try to think of all the details. How old were you? What were you wearing? Where were you? Do you remember what was happening before the moment? How did you handle the feeling? How does it compare to the story of your earliest memory?

- Awareness of your loneliness can be a signal that something needs to change. What might your guess be as to what the change would be? Besides your loneliness, what else in your life feels uncomfortable? Take time throughout your day to notice your twinges of discomfort and write them down. Do this for a week. Notice the common themes of your discomfort.

What You Tell Your Yourself

Increase your resilience by focusing on the ways in which you can tackle your worries in small steps that will help you feel better and focus your attention towards solutions.

Instead of Saying This	Try Saying This
I can't believe I made that mistake. I am so stupid.	How can I do this better next time?

Instead of Saying This	Try Saying This
I just don't understand this math. Why am I the only one in the class who doesn't get this?	I don't understand this. What do I need to do to get the help I need to understand this?
Why don't they like me?	What are the qualities that I am looking for in a friend? What can I do to attract those qualities. In myself and in those around me?
I hate myself for eating all of this food. I am a fat pig with no self-control.	I am disappointed in my choice to overeat. What do I need to do right now to feel better about my body right now. What is one strategy I can take to do this differently for the next time?
I totally lost my patience with my son. I am a terrible dad.	I recognize that I lost my patience with my son. I said things I should not have. What can I do to repair harm and have a better relationship with my son?

Routines and Repetition

What are the ways you can make repetition work for you?

- Start with morning and evening routines.
- Pick two or three activities that you want to incorporate in your routine. Start with ten-minute blocks of time.

- Get to a place of discomfort, but not so uncomfortable that it takes up all of your brainpower and willpower to complete it.

- Honour your successes. Reward your effort, not your skill. In perseverance training, the effort is more important than the skill.

- Do what you can to make it easy. Enlist a friend. Tell those who will encourage your goal about your efforts, or do the work when you are most likely to complete the task.

- Imagine your future self. What will it feel like to have all your credit cards paid off? What will it be like to be able to swim across the lake? What will it be like to complete your goals?

- Be your own cheerleader. Talk to yourself in ways that focus on success. Your "head" can be your most effective self-saboteur if you let it. It can also be your strongest supporter. Train your brain to focus on where you WANT to go, not where you are AFRAID to be.

- Every time you strengthen your perseverance skills, every time you practice consistency in the tasks that you want to accomplish, you are teaching all the people around you. What you do and do repeatedly is what you teach. Model perseverance and see the community around you inspired by your efforts.

Finish Tasks to the End

- Find your unfinished projects.

- Which ones do you need to ditch and which ones do you need to complete?

- Make a list.

- Go through all of your loose ends and tackle them one by one.

- It could be something as simple as repairing a creaky floorboard, or getting to that half-finished art project you started a year ago. Or maybe it is about completing the divorce paperwork, or concluding that difficult conversation you started with your boss.

- Celebrate each completion. It could be communicating your success to an accountability partner, extra time on a task you love to do, or a small treat or purchase. Celebrating your completions will help your body remember how good it feels to get the task done and will provide further incentive for tackling goals in the future.

Chapter Five
Transformation

---

*Communion is mutual trust, mutual belonging; it is the
to-and-fro movement of love between two people where
each one gives and each one receives. Communion is not
a fixed state; it is an ever-growing and deepening reality
that can turn sour if one person tries to possess the
other, thus preventing growth. Communion is mutual
vulnerability and openness one to the other.*

Jean Vanier

*When you change the way you look at things,
things you look at change.* **Max Plank**

It Isn't Pretty, But It's Success

IT IS SUNDAY MORNING and I am with my running
group, training for a marathon. It is early morning and

already it is too hot. Our pace group gathers and I am fearful at the thought of our impending long run. Sixteen miles in the hot sun feels less like a challenge and more like a trial. But when the going gets tough, our pace group cracks jokes – The cornier the better. "Why is Peter Pan always flying? Because he never lands!" "What did the tree say to the wind? Leaf me alone!" "Why did the cookie go to the hospital? Because he felt crummy!" The banter starts off strong, but after a few hills, the chatter falls silent and we plod through the miles. The sweat has dried on my body, leaving streaks of dried salt along my face and arms. We keep going. As we head towards the final stretch, the banter picks up. "What do you call a pony with a little cough? A little hoarse!" "How do you make friends with a squirrel? You act like a nut!" We are heading up the final hill towards the finish line. There is no shade and my pace cuts to a crawl. At the end of the run, we are all tired and smelly. One of the runners turns to look at the group and he says, "It isn't pretty, but it's success."

And so, sticky with salt, drenched in sweat, we stretch out our legs. We head for the showers, careful to clean off all the evidence of the challenging run. But our muscles, our heart, our lungs and our legs will not forget. They will remember this run, and the next time heat, struggle and hardship come, they will remember. We survived this one and we will survive the next one - and the next one and the next.

Life by a Thousand Efforts

Since that gruelling run in the scorching sun, I have often used the line, "It isn't pretty, but it's success," to describe the moments when achievement looks less like receiving an Academy Award and more like being dragged through mud. Sometimes success will feel uncomfortable, unfinished and less than satisfying.

Entering into suffering that comes from the radical and painful interruption of crisis will be difficult, but it is also brings compassion, awareness and joy. As you enter suffering, use the tools that you have to support yourself. Trust that some kind of transformation is waiting for you on the other side. Struggle teaches your cells how to adapt, evolve and grow stronger. This is one of the fundamental opportunities that crisis brings into your life.

Crisis allows you the opportunity to fully participate in your life. When you are training your brain to look at joy rather than settle into despair, you choose to make small, repeated efforts that will bring you towards joy, even if your efforts require you to enter into more suffering. It is life by a thousand efforts. Some of these efforts will appear enormous - like burying your child, or learning to unravel post-traumatic stress. Yet ultimately, every life-giving decision comes down to small, repeated acts, completed thousands of time, which, over time, become ingrained in your consciousness, in your day to day practice and in your natural way of being.

Life by a thousand efforts means that every day, you choose to take small repeated steps that bring you freedom, joy and contentment. Ultimately, it is the small steps that help you work through the big explosions of feelings that occur during a crisis. When you choose to allow crisis to move through you and then past you, you experience transformation. Every time you practiced a disruption, you have taken a small step towards challenging your box of fear. You expand your vision of what is possible. Once you have chosen to explore what it means to live outside the box that says, "I am safe." You expand your world. You evolve your courage to move through the fear and you find out what lies on the other side.

What You Want Wants You

Change doesn't happen in a vacuum. Your desire for a bigger life is part of a series of events and experiences that bring you to that desire. Perhaps it has been brewing for generations. Crisis transforms you and your surrounding community from the inside out. Every change, no matter how small, impacts the surrounding environments. A shoe transforms to the shape of the foot - but the foot has also transformed the shoe. Change informs ALL interactions you have with the world around you.

You have the ability to connect stories and experiences that align with your freedom. When you put energy towards your wants and desires, the world around you conspires to help you move towards them. Your wants and desires are also things. They have a weight and a mass that interact with the world around you. The advantage of transforming one area of your life is that pretty soon, you will want balance in all parts of your life. You will want to streamline the number of hours you work, so that you have balance in your home and personal life. You will desire movement if you lead a sedentary life, more silence if your life is noisy, more silliness if your life is too serious.

You will find that the things that you used to put up with will no longer be tolerable. As you allow crisis to transform your life, the deep and committed relationships in your life will also stretch, expand and shift towards a new balance. This might take some adjustment, but in the end, every small change you make moves you closer towards your transformation. You will find a greater ease in speaking to your strengths, as well as to your vulnerabilities. All of your small or big leaps into the unknown provide you with the confidence to speak to your present experience and share it with your loved ones. And they will do the same for you. You will experience the, "To and fro movement of love."

You are not alone in your healing. You are not the only one who desires your transformation. What you want, wants you.

Small Boxes of Fear

A client in my energy medicine practice was overcome with grief. Her adult child no longer wanted to be a part of her life. She had spent over 22 years caring for and providing resources for her son. She raised him as a single parent and made tremendous sacrifices over the years in order to support his passion for competitive motocross racing. Years later, as she found herself recovering from a significant car accident, her son was not helping her in her recovery. Instead, he was distant and disconnected. Slowly she was able to see how her desire to make her son's life easier than her own, meant he did not get the practice to handle uncomfortable feelings. He also did not get the practice of helping his mother and working to contribute to their shared home.

So often you think that you can *do* your way out of a situation. You try to work harder. In many cases, you find yourself in the midst of unbalance and you think the way to level the scales is by giving to those around you. I see this happen all the time in my practice with parents who strive to provide as many benefits to their children as they possibly can, intent that their children will avoid the suffering or hardship that they themselves received as children. But in all of this giving, they restrict the opportunities for their children to practice giving. This sets up an expectation that receiving without giving is normal. It becomes an expectation that 'others' are responsible to take care of their uncomfortable feelings. This sense of entitlement disadvantages a young brain. You pass down the imbalance and practice required to both give and receive. Living in imbalanced states can bring negative consequences for both over givers and over receivers.

Parents, caregivers and "over givers" can inadvertently shield their children, clients and loved ones from the practice they need to develop the skills necessary to manage conflict, crisis and well-being. We all need the practice of giving, gratitude and daily responsibilities. When we don't get this practice, we are not developing the habits and skills required to grow resilience, stress management and courage. Empathy is a skill. It needs to be practiced. The idea of forgoing your needs or your comforts over the needs of someone else requires repeated effort.

You can pass on your fears and anxieties to your children. In my role as an elementary school counsellor, I see how wounds and unresolved felt experiences inform how we teach and treat others. In many cases, parents try to protect their children from the painful childhood traumas that happened to them. They may inadvertently teach their children to avoid their fear. The protected children get limited practice with stress, failure and problem solving. The very skills and experiences required to develop resilience and confidence do not get practiced and so, they become fearful children.

You don't want children and loved ones to avoid pain. You want them to have the skills and the confidence to manage their suffering and to know that they have the capacity to change that suffering into growth and transformation. Everyone needs practice at making mistakes, taking risks and failing. Managing suffering or discomfort allows us the practice of experiencing success, developing confidence and learning to take responsibility. We can all benefit from opportunities to live life out of our small boxes of fear.

Relationships are about supporting growth, independence and well-being. When you find yourself hovering over loved ones, pay attention to who you are trying to help. Is this about your fear? Or is this about supporting your children in being independent, strong and well? If you feel yourself giving more then you are receiving, this is a sign that you are projecting your fear and your responsibilities onto someone else.

One of the ways that you can work towards recalibrating the balance is to ensure that you make it known that you require gratitude for your efforts and thoughtfulness. It is especially important that the people closest to you are taught to say please and thank you, and that you expect gratitude for the work that you and others do. As part of their membership to families and communities, everyone should have responsibilities and tasks.

Love, done well, needs to move. Relationships need to flow, move, arrive, return, respond and then move again. It is about the active connection between two forms of energy and people, pets, plants and food are all energy.

When we constantly give, we are missing out on the 'to and fro movement of love' that Vanier writes about. Relationships are designed to support growth, independence and wellness. When you try to fix the lives of people that you care about, you are teaching them to avoid self-responsibility. Imbalanced energy will weaken the relationship, and left unattended, may even contribute to the breakdown of the relationship. Provide opportunities to both give and receive every day. Everybody has work to do and we all have opportunities to receive from each other. As you evolve past your crisis, be prepared to continue to navigate the 'to and fro movement of love' in your meaningful relationships.

The Long View

Another way to help you to change your story is to think about how the changes and difficult choices you make today will affect your life farther off in the distance. It is hard to see how the end of your marriage today can bring you joy, but what will the ending of an unhealthy marriage look like five years down the road? What will it look like in ten years? The benefit of taking the long view is being studied in all kinds of disciplines; marketing, medicine, education, even climate change. Increasingly, we as a culture are not just examining the quick and easy fix, but also, the solution that creates the biggest benefits for the long haul.

This strategy has been a tremendous help to me during many of my crisis moments. Several years ago, I invested a significant amount of my resources with someone I believed was taking care of my financial investments. At some point, my sister and some close friends began to get suspicious, and began to carefully scrutinize the investments, only to find substantial mishandling of my investments. I had to face some significant financial losses and admit to some poor financial choices and partnerships, one of the thoughts that helped me move forward was to think about myself, not just in the present moment, but in five years from now. It helped me to not just focus on my present-day woes, but to look at what I could achieve five, or ten years from now. Instead of just seeing loss, the long view helped me see how my present day, painful choices could be an investment in my future self. By acknowledging my learning and losses, I also could appreciate how the lessons I learned from the experience could help me make financial gains for my future self. When I took the perspective of the long view, I could see how difficult choices today would help me build a more solid financial stability in the long run. Holding the long view and understanding that the pain I was experiencing would look very different five years from now, helped me to move forward and take the necessary painful steps to work on my solution.

Ask yourself the same question in relation to your own problems: how can I be present in this crisis so that it will make me stronger? How will the way I handle this crisis today, make me a better and stronger person, one year from now? Five years from now? Ten years from now? When you choose to stay present in your wounded felt experiences, understanding that your present suffering is a result of repairing, restoring and healing, then you have an opportunity to experience transformation.

If you do this well, it is a small leap. It is not a big, overwhelming impossible step. It is a natural progression. Your small and big efforts will acclimatize you to a new and healthy "normal." The work you put into examining your crisis, healing your old stories, and training your brain and body to develop new, healthy habits will set you up for success. You can now imagine yourself as a confident, free, capable and resilient person and better yet, you have the skills and strength to live with capacity, confidence and freedom.

This is your new story. If you have the courage to embrace your crisis, if you enter into your suffering, and receive it, then you transmute it into something that moves you into your new story. A crisis done well, leads to suffering. Suffering leads you to opportunities to enter your healing. Healing allows you to find the story that must die. Death leaves a space for a new story to arise. Living the new story brings you to your transformation. You can experience the freedom to leave an unhealthy relationship and you also have to responsibility to deal with the emptiness and loss. When you face your crisis, you will start to recognize the arrival of your new story. It is the beginning of coming back to you.

Death Is Not the End

This next point may not be everyone's cup of tea but it is still something worth considering. It is my point of view that some form of you continues long after your body dies. Your legacy on earth is not just your past, but it is also the energy you leave behind in electrical form. You might call this spirit, or guardian angels or ghosts. In my energy medicine practice I sometimes get to see or hear them as they work in some way to assist the session. I am acutely aware that some form of life continues outside our physical form. For me, this requires every human being to take responsibility for actions and choices well past the death of their bodies. Your life does not end when you die.

Think about how you behave *now* and what you learn *now* as being able to affect your future 'electrical self'. Think about what is going to happen after you die and become one of those electrical beings. Do you want to continue to affect positive change? Your work does not end when your body hits the ground. You keep going. And you have to think about the generation that follows you, the 10th generation that follows you and even the 1000th generation that follows you. Take the long view, because how you behave now will affect the choices that you have, the potential that you have, once you become all of that electricity. You take on another form and continue evolving. Power comes in looking at the long view. And the long view goes far beyond the timeline of your body. Crisis gives you a hint of that long view.

I think about the children that I will be the guardian angel of thousands of generations to come. I think about the world that I leave; not just for my nieces and nephews and their children, but I think of their children's children and the children of their children. I want to leave this world in the best way that I possibly can, sowing seeds that will last long after my body's lifetime, that will foster a life of balance for those that will come after me. This is your loving legacy when you do crisis well.

What Can I Do to Continue My Transformation?

In this final chapter, we will look at several strategies that can support you in moving forward in your transformation. The idea is to notice your big uncomfortable feelings. Or you notice that you keep having the same arguments over and over. Or you notice that you are tired of your addictions and distractions or that you are just plain tired of your constant exhausted.

You are going to need practice at holding your success. The actions you take on a daily basis, in thought, action and attitude, will build the foundation for your stronger, more resilient and more capable self. Find activities that resonate, or feel easy or doable. Build repetition. Take your time in developing routines, as you will be practicing these habits for a lifetime. When you are ready, add additional habits. Slow and steady wins the race.

Prepare for Success

The PreMortem is a concept developed by Gary Klein, a research psychologist who studied decision making especially as it pertained in business. His research showed that one of the greatest predictors of a successful project was determined by what organizations did *before* the event. He discovered that companies that planned for failure and then problem solved solutions were consistently more successful. Preparing for failure is a strong predictor of success.

You can practice the PreMortem concept in your own life by planning your activities ahead of time and troubleshooting potential problems. This is a great tactic to use in everyday life. It is especially useful for your morning routine. The more you pre-plan to make the most stressful times of your day as easy as possible, the more you set up your day for success.

A PreMortem means that you organize your day, event, stressful social encounter, or financial plan, prior to the event. It means you set your morning up the night before. Take the time to carefully go through your plan for the day: double-check to make sure you have everything you need, the nutrition, money, paperwork, gas in the car, the attitude, the right clothing – whatever elements you need to make your day run smoothly. Plan to get to your event early. Plan for backup systems should technology fail. Rehearse and anticipate potential problems.

Help your brain organize and anticipate problems. Find an area in your life that you want to set up for success. It could be your mornings, a less fractious relationship with your teenage daughter, your finances, your fitness program, or an innovative pilot project you want to implement at work. Break down the day in small bites and implement the PreMortem.

Show Up

In our modern world that is increasingly reliant on technology for interaction, there are limited experiences of eye contact, human touch, communication, and play. Yet as we have already discussed in previous chapters, our bodies evolved with millions of experiences of connection, touch, and engagement. We need contact and engagement with others. A baby that has not been touched will have permanent cognitive impairment. Babies that are held and receive lots of human contact develop more receptors to read stress and will be better able to shut off stress. When we are children, play, in particular, unstructured play, helps us to rehearse and practice healthy social engagement. It provides us with tools to read social cues, learn and practice social norms, practice delayed gratification and empathy. Without the repeated physical experience of others, you will have less ability to manage your feelings.

Look up. Try to make eye contact with those around you. Say thank you, notice what is happening around you and acknowledge people's presence. Create small, consistent opportunities to engage with the people around you. All of these encounters add up. Increase the human contact that your body receives. Hugs play a significant role in well-being, contentment and rest.   Human contact improves math skills, decreases pain and increases group performance. The ability to give and receive eye contact, loving human touch, hugs and social connections are critical in lifelong brain development.

Be Kind

On one of my Sunday training runs, we were scheduled to run an 18-mile route. It was hot, humid and I wasn't feeling well. Early on in the run, I felt myself lagging, and I was at the back of the pack on every hill. When we took a break for water, I told Al, my run leader, that I might not finish the run. He didn't seem to hear me. He grabbed my hand and said, "You are coming with me", and before I could say anything, he brought me to the front of the group and ran alongside me. I finished all eighteen miles without injury or pain. Al's decision to share his energy and confidence with me gave me the opportunity to finish the training run. On my own, I would have quit.

Al's kindness helped me, but it also helped Al. He received the same benefits of support, resilience and strength that he provided for me. Kindness works a lot like TOMS shoes slogan; Get One, Give One. TOMS shoes started with the idea of creating a business model that embedded a product with the act of helping others. The founder, Blake Mycoskie created a successful business model that matched every shoe purchase with a free pair of shoes for a child in need. Practicing acts of kindness gives you a boost – giving, volunteering, sharing your time and talents provides you with hits of the feel good chemical dopamine. It helps you increase your feeling of well-being. You practice thinking about others. It supports you in getting perspective about your own worries as you get the habit of seeing beyond yourself and looking at the big picture. It helps you create connections and community. Kindness and being of service works on others, but it also works on you too.

Have Less

Humans evolved by living outdoors seeing wide-open spaces and having few possessions. It is astounding to think that during all of our many years on this planet that it has only been 30,000 years since we started settling and creating communities that farmed and bred animals. Before that, we relied on very few things.

Our brains and our bodies are not used to accumulating so much stuff. In the last one hundred years, we have seen an explosion of the accumulation of things. But all of this clutter affects the way you think. It increases anxiety. It creates more choices and more decisions. It amplifies the number of responsibilities you hold. It has its own kind of weight. In my energy medicine practice, evidence of too much clutter shows up in many of my client's energy fields. I understand this battle, as I struggle with this myself. It has been a challenge to try and simplify my own life.

Take steps to minimize the things that you own. Let go of the stuff that you don't really need, or that serves no purpose. Think carefully about what you *really* need and then take the steps to eliminate the clutter. Clearing space in your environment helps you sleep and calms you down. It ultimately helps you live more simply with less opportunities for crisis.

What You DO Have

There is a reason why gratitude lists have grown in popularity. Focusing on what you DO have is good for you. It trains you to spotlight your perspective on what is working for you. It trains you to think about solutions. When you think about what is working, your body chemistry changes for the better. It leaves you in a better position to solve a problem, rather than stay in it. Gratitude is like a sturdy rope that gets dropped down to you when you are in your pit of pitifulness. It is a lifeline. If you write down your gratitude, you are further anchoring the information and the experience in your brain.

Create an Electronic Free Time Zone

A twelve-year-old girl sits across from me in my counselling office. I have asked her to describe last night's activities in her home. After she completed her homework she headed to her room to watch her favourite YouTube channels. After finishing his homework, her 14-year-old brother retreated to his room to plays video games. Her dad settled in downstairs and watched TV. Her mom was upstairs in her bedroom, connecting online with family and friends. All this private electronic screen time is quickly becoming the 'new normal' in North American homes. It prevents the repeated experience of human contact, face-to-face recognition and self regulation skills that our brain and body require to develop and strengthen.

Our biology requires common experiences with other humans. We have chemical responses that favour human connection. We have spent millions of years surviving in tribes. When you are around people who care about you, it affects your body's ability to stay calm, digest food, breathe slower, feel relaxed, think clearly, make better decisions and heal faster. Human connection improves our ability to regulate our feelings. It provides you with practice in social engagement. It is the tiny small nuances of human interaction, repeated thousands of times that inform your body. These small bits of information teach your brain how to get along with others, take care of your big feelings and work in collectives.

In recent years, the advancement of technology and the explosion of digital use provides us with the opportunity to distract ourselves every second of the day. But these quick distractions take a toll on our brains. By engaging with and relying on technology so heavily it does not allow us the practice of connecting with others - or even with our own thoughts. Start by giving yourself a thirty-minute window where you don't look at your email, or any of your digital devices. Instead of tuning the world out through digital distractions, go for a walk, or hang out with someone. Or you can sit in connection with others, or in solitude and be still. Choose to live a small part of your day in the absence of digital media. Perhaps you can take it further by picking one day of the week where you stay away from technology altogether. Find your day of rest and notice the effects it has on your mood, your energy levels and your communication with others.

Heavy Labour

Lifting weights or engaging in heavy manual labour calms your body. Again, this goes back to how we evolved – living outdoors, walking, looking for food sources, avoiding predators and contributing to a tribe. Physical labour was a routine part of our daily lives. Heavy labour regulates your feelings and helps provide you with perspective and clarity. Lifting, pushing, pulling and moving heavy objects allows your body to release cortisol and adrenaline. It temporarily shifts your worries onto the immediate task. This has a calming effect on the body. You may have already noticed this when you let off steam by washing windows, cleaning out a closet or doing some vigorous housework. Physical labour also provides a natural way for you to eliminate stress and excess energy. It has the added benefit of increasing muscle mass and improving overall fitness.

Get Bored

Studies indicate that boredom increases creativity, provides opportunities to be self-reflective and can reduce stress. It also gives you practice at regulating your feelings and mood. Schedule time in your life where you actively do nothing. Don't watch TV, eat, smoke, drink or sleep -

just do nothing. Breathe; listen to the chatter of your brain, your to-do list, your self-talk and do nothing. Allow yourself the opportunity to get quiet and calm. Being comfortable with boredom might take a bit of time. The idea of of doing nothing, even for just ten minutes, without any stimulation or escapes can be anxiety provoking but if you can practice this consistently, you will get to experience the magic of stillness, creativity and a calm mind.

Recap

Transformation happens in small repeated practices. It is life by a thousand efforts. If you avoid your suffering and your crisis, you risk passing it down to your children. Take the long view. The discomfort and pain of creating new habits and staying with your felt experiences will make huge changes for your future self, which continues even after your body leaves this earth. Some of the small daily habits that will help your transformation include: taking time to plan for setbacks and setting up your day for success, showing up, practicing eye contact, play and connecting with others, being kind to others, having less and eliminating clutter, practicing gratitude, creating an electronic free zone, lifting weights or participating in manual labour and giving yourself opportunities to be bored.

What You Can Do

Hold the Long View

Reflect on the following questions:

- How can I be present in this crisis so that it will make me stronger?

- How will the way I handle this crisis today, make me a better and stronger person one year from now? Five years? Ten years?

Prepare for Success

- Help your brain organize and anticipate problems. Find an area in your life that you want to set up for success. It could be your mornings, a less fractious relationship with your teenage daughter, your finances, your fitness program, or an innovative pilot project you want to implement at work.

- Determine actions required to create success.

- List possible problems that might get in the way of the success.

- Brainstorm ways in which you can solve the problem. If you are unsure of what you need to do, consult with experts or support systems.

- Break down the day in small activities.

- Create lists based on the small activities.

- Review the lists and complete the activities outlined in the list.

Show Up

- Give your time and talent. Explore the opportunities available in your community that are a good fit for your interests and skillset.

- When you are having a conversation with someone, give them your complete attention. Put your phone out of eyesight, face the speaker with your body and be fully present in the conversation.

- Have scheduled, focused time with meaningful relationships.

- Eat meals with others.

- Increase opportunities for loving touch. Get regular massages, increase sexual contact and intimacy with your partner, join a dance class, spend time and contact with pets – These are all great ways to increase opportunities for loving touch in your life.

Be Kind

- Choose to do one kind thing for someone close to you. It could be completing a chore that they do not like doing, writing a note of appreciation, purchasing a small gift, giving them your undistracted attention, finding a way to support them in a goal, participating in an activity they enjoy, or letting them know what you appreciate about them.

- Write a small note of appreciation to someone who has demonstrated kindness to you in the past few days.

- Phone someone who you haven't spoken to lately, ask questions and listen.

- Complete one random act of kindness anonymously. Write a note of encouragement to someone at work, or buy someone a coffee or tea.

Have Less

- Tackle one space at a time, e.g. a sock drawer, kitchen cupboard or entrance closet. Consider eliminating all of the items you no longer use, either by throwing them out, giving them away or donating them to a second-hand store.

- Have a friend or someone you trust come and support you in making the decisions.

- Consider selling items through eBay, Craigs List or a garage sale.

- Eliminate 50% of everything in one room like a guest bedroom or bathroom. Spend time in the space, getting used to living and using a space that feels "empty". Notice what shows up with your feelings and memories while spending time in the clutter free space. This will provide you with your own personal observations about what emotional wounds exist underneath all the clutter. Seek professional support in tackling these emotional wounds, which can be significant.

- Consider using resources to help you on your quest, such as Marie Kondo's book, *The Life Changing Magic of Tidying Up.* Commit to completing the "Kondo Method" in clearing your space of items that no longer serve you. In her book, she describes a process where you touch every item and decide if the item should be kept or eliminated.

What You Do Have

- Keep a gratitude journal. Write down three things that happened during your day that you are grateful for. Write down one thing that you are least grateful for.

- Write down three things in your life that you are grateful for. Share your gratitude with another person and listen to yourself sharing your gratitude out loud.

- In the evening, write five statements about your day framed around capacity and strength. For example, *I don't like that I yelled at my husband before dinner, but I noticed that I was able to quickly catch what I was doing, name it and change the tone so that we had a good interaction. I am glad I could complete the first 20 minutes of the fitness program. I appreciate the fact that I was able to talk to three of my co-workers and I engaged in a positive and conscious social interaction.*

- Notice the inner dialogue that you have throughout the day. What are the times of the day when the inner dialogue turns negative or impatient? Is it at the end of the day, when you are hungry, when you have been sitting for too long, when you are stressed? What can you do to change the conditions so that you can focus on success?

- Rewrite positive inner dialogue scripts that can counteract your challenging moments. Examples include:

  - *I recognize that I am tired and hungry and I know I have the capacity to take care of myself until I can eat and rest.*

  - *I am capable of speaking my opinions in a respectful way.*

  - *I don't have to have the approval of my boss to be successful. I am going to be okay. I am okay right now.*

- I can be a loving parent, while still holding a firm boundary with my teenage daughter.

- It is okay for me to make mistakes. I can learn from them and do better. I am more than my mistakes.

Create an Electronic Free Time Zone

- Find a time that you can consistently be with others. Before, during and after the main meal is a good place to start.

- Make all meal times electronic free zones.

- Find activities to do together such as, playing a board game, going for a walk, listening to a podcast or story.

- Try activities or hobbies that you are interested in exploring.

- Complete household or routine chores.

Heavy Labour

- Consider adding weight training to your fitness regime. Tim Ferriss in *The Four-Hour Body* suggests that even 75 kettlebell swings, 2-3 times a week will make a considerable impact on physical fitness.

- Include one chore every day that provides you with an opportunity to practice physical manual labour – washing floors, toilets, or the car are all good examples.

- Include a 10-minute high intensity or Tabata work-out sometime in your day. YouTube links are included in the chapter notes.

- When you are overwhelmed, frustrated or anxious, a three minute high intensity activity can help you shift your energy and change your mood, as well as provide you with the ability to focus your attention. Some examples are:

  - go outside and do three 40 second sprints with a 20 second recovery in between sprints,

  - complete 10 sit-ups, 10 push ups and 10 burpees, (increase to 15, then 20 when you are ready),

  - climb up and down stairs, or touch your head, your waist, your knees and your toes for three minutes.

Get Bored

- Schedule time to disconnect from all electronic stimulation including TV, podcasts, social media and news feeds.

- Avoid eating or drinking while you are "doing nothing."

- Go for a walk, or hang out in your room. Listen to music. Take ten minutes to do nothing.

Epilogue

A CRISIS DONE WELL leads to suffering. It is the answer to your prayer. Crisis is your invitation to change an old story that no longer serves you. You get to decide whether you want to keep the story, or choose another one. Either way, you will suffer. When you choose the better feeling story, you can convert the suffering into your transformation. Love and connection require you to practice and expect others to both give and receive. Take the long view. Your life is greater than the experiences you have in your body. When you choose to heal your life and focus on your courage and resilience, you impact your present and the future, for many generations to come. You are not alone in your healing. What you want, wants you. Fear is easy. It lets you protect your vulnerability and your ugly. Remember it is about taking small steps. Steps that feel true to you. Repeat them, over time. Focus on where you want to go. This is life by a thousand efforts.

Finishing

And here we are: right back at the spot where we began. You've learned that the full circle of crisis is much bigger than you and your old stories. You've learned that the seeds of the crisis started before you arrived in your body. You've learned that every crisis started as a series of conflicts that were not acknowledged. You can now appreciate that all your feelings provide you with vital information – information that is critical in helping you to live a fuller and better life. You are now able to accept the responsibility of taking care of your feelings, conflicts and your crisis. You have learned how to disrupt your old story. You have learned how you can choose to enter into your crisis, to pause, go slow, listen and be still. You now know you must allow your felt experiences to transform your suffering. You are now able to use your disruptions to slowly change the old story that crisis insists you shatter, and you can practice life by a thousand efforts. You breathe this in, and show up in your life and stay present.

Home

You probably don't even recognize you are back where you started. Everything is the same and yet, everything completely transformed. It is not the landscape that has changed – It is you. You have lost the old story so you are lighter. You are not carrying all that weight that did not belong to you. You have experienced yourself receiving risks and taking risks. You have witnessed your dying's and you have witnessed your transformations. You have practiced meeting your fear. You have worked at finding community, taking the long view, framing your challenges and more. Hopefully, you are a little stronger, more patient and resilient. You are able to stay still, get bored and listen to others. All your small repeated transformational habits have changed the world around you.

I cannot leave you without thanking you for the privilege of being your companion as you have worked through your crisis. It was an honour to be present to your brokenness. It was my delight to share your courage and it was my joy to see you hold your transformation. I am leaving, but please remember that you are never alone. The entire world conspires with you to guide you to your heart's desire.

Happy travels. All is well.

If you want to learn more about the ideas discussed in this book, or if you would like to contact me, you can check out my website. Chapter notes and further research, links and worksheets can be found on http://creativeedge-consulting.com

CPSIA information can be obtained
at www.ICGtesting.com
Printed in the USA
LVHW04s2130300418
575467LV00002B/2/P